The Proper RULES for FASTING!

(The Complete Instruction Manual for True Repentance!)

By
The Worldwide People's Revolution!®

Book 046 ♥

(The Cover Photo shows an Unclean Man)

Copyright, Dedication and Introduction

By
Dr. Samuel Walker Edison, Ph.D, MA, BS, and QC!

ISBN — 13: 978-1541-3906-69
ISBN — 10: 1541-3906-60

00-02 [_] No Portion of this Inspired Book shall be Reproduced by any Means for Sale without Written Permission from **The Worldwide People's Revolution!®** However, with our Permission, anyone in the World is Free to Reproduce Exact Copies, and Sell them for a Reasonable Profit, and KEEP 90% of the Net Profits for themselves: beCause **"The Swanky Associations of Working Soldiers"** only Want 10% of the Net Profits for the Construction of: **"The Great World TEMPLE of PEACE,"** which will Hopefully be Constructed in Jerusalem, which will be the Tallest and Largest Building in the World, being nearly a Mile Tall and 8+ Miles in Diameter, being a Dodecagon with 12 Sides, in 60 Great Stone Terraces, with 6 shorter Stone Terraces within each Great Terrace, which Temple will Contain the Headquarters for **"The New RIGHTEOUS One-World Government,"** whose Beautiful Stone Dome Homes will be Built within those Small Terraces, each of which will be about 60 feet Tall, having Gardens, Vineyards, and Orchards Planted on the Roofs of the Stone Dome Homes, where the Elected Officials will Live with their Staffs and their Voluntary Servants, who will Attend to their Gardens, Cooking, House Cleaning, and so, in Exchange for getting to Live there, who may also Eat whatever they Want to at the **Royal Swanky Buffets** throughout the Great Temple, or Devote themselves to **Swanky Fasting Sanitariums** within the Great Temple, which will be Open to all Visitors who have Filled Out and Filed on the Internet **"The Complete SURVEYS of our VALUES!"** (SURVEYS of Religious Spiritual Political Governmental Sexual Social

Moral Economic Business Labor Habitual and Miscellaneous VALUES!) By The Worldwide People's Revolution!®, Book 059, which all Elected Officials will also have to Fill Out and File on the Internet, BEFORE they can be Elected: so that we Electors can Know for a Fact WHO we are Electing, and WHY: beCause we are Sick of Voting for Dimwitcrats and Reprobates who cannot be Trusted.

00-03 [_] So, O Doctor Edison, it Sounds as if **"The Great World TEMPLE of PEACE"** will be much more than just the Headquarters for **"The New RIGHTEOUS One-World Government,"** whose Elected Officials must be HOLY MEN, huh? {See www.Amazon.com for: **"HOW to Become a HOLY Man!" (40 Good Reasons WHY People Should FAST and PRAY!) By The Worldwide People's Revolution!®** Book 045.}

00-04 [_] Well, that Great Temple will be a Good Example in several Ways. For Example,

> A-[_] The Building, itself, will be a Good Example for the Construction of ALL **"GLORIOUS Swanky Hotels Castles and Fortresses!" (Beautiful Planned City States for WISE Intelligent Well-Educated People with Common Sense and Good Understanding!) By The Worldwide People's Revolution!®**, Book 019, which will also be Built in Great Terraces, whereby neither Automobiles nor any other Stinking Noisy Capitalist Abominations will be Needed nor Wanted: beCause of Using Electric Elevators, Escalators, and Electric Subway Trains for Transportation. Indeed, that Great Temple will Contain Beautiful Stone Dome Home Complexes, the likes of which everyone in the World may Inherit, if they are Willing and Able to Help Build them, which Means that they must also be Willing and Able to LEARN and WORK: beCause there are NO "Freebies," as they say, except for those People who are too Old, too Young, too Sick, too Disabled, or too Mentally Challenged to Help with the Construction, who will most Certainly be Provided with Good Places to Live, if they are Cooperative, and also Answer the Questions in **"The Complete SURVEYS of our VALUES,"** whereby we might Understand WHERE they Belong within the Swanky Fortress System. After all, it is Obvious that none of those Sick Degenerated People would QUALIFY for any Positions within **"The New RIGHTEOUS One-World Government!" (HOW to Establish a Righteous One-World Government without Going to WAR!) By The Worldwide People's Revolution!®** Book 056.

> B-[_] Secondly, that Great Temple will be Inhabited with Elected Officials who have done a LOT of Fasting and Praying, whereby their Brains are Functioning Correctly with a Capital C, whereby much Time and Energy will be Saved on the Construction of MILLIONS of those **"GLORIOUS Swanky Hotels Castles and Fortresses,"** which are Designed for LIVING, and NOT for the Profit of a few Greedy Rich Hogs: beCause True Prosperity for the Masses of People is the Primary Goal for Building them. However, when we say, "NOT for Profit," we Specifically Mean not for the Profit of Lying Red Jew CAPITALISTS — such as those Greedy SELFISH Red Jews on Wall Street in New Yuck City, who have Raked in TRILLIONS of Dollars by Means of their Money Games, while Billions of People in this World of Woes are Suffering without Fresh Clean Air to Breathe, Pure Living Water to Drink, Wholesome Natural Foods to Eat, nor Secure Spacious Stone Dome Homes to Live in, which have Home-craft Workshops with Well-

3

made Tools, Sales Shops, 4 Large one-half-million-gallon Swanky Cisterns for Water Storage, and one-acre Gardens for all Families — "Straight" or GAY, you might say — who will be Happy and most Satisfied to do their Gardening According to: **"The LUSCIOUS All-Mineral Organic Method of Gardening!" (HOW to Grow DELICIOUS Satisfying Foods for Potential Kingz and Kweenz in Swanky PALACES!)**, Book 021: beCause of being Sick of **"Poverty Hunger Riots Strikes Brutalities Election Deceptions and Civil Wars!" (The High Price that we Earthlings have Paid for Leaving the Good Land!)** Book 014. {See www.Amazon.com for: **"Are we Tax Slaves of a Lower Order than Lying Red JEWS?" (HOW to be Liberated from all Slavery, Worldwide!)**, Book 052, plus: **"The Great False Economy is now DEBUNKED!" (Adolf Hitler had a much Better Economic System!)**, Book 053, plus: **"The UGLY Scarred Dishonest Face of Poor Old Miserable UNCLE SAM!" (A Memorial Day Legacy!) By The Worldwide People's Revolution!®** Book 054.}

C-[ ] Thirdly, **"The Great World TEMPLE of PEACE"** will be Representing ALL Peoples in the World, and not just **"The Divided States of United Lies!" (The so-called "United States of North America" in Disguise!)**, Book 058, whose Head of Lies will be Thoroughly Removed from the Chief Snake by **"The Swanky Sword of Divine Truths!" (The Most Powerful Weapon in the Whole Universe!) By The Worldwide People's Revolution!®** Book 067. Yes, that Babylonian System of Massive Confusion is otherwise known in Biblical Terms as *"The Economic System of the Dragon, who Speaks like an Innocent Lamb, and Acts like a Snake, which has 2 Little Political Horns, which Appear to Butt Against each other, being 2 Different Sides of the same Coin, you might say,"* which are otherwise known as the Democrats and Republicans, who have no Reasonable Solutions for anything! Indeed, they Work Hand-in-Hand with the Lying Zionist Red Jew Bankers' Military Industrial Drug-pushers' Congressional News Media Hollywood Bankers' Complex: beCause those Lying Zionist Red Jews are the Puppet Masters, who Control the Money Supply, and thus Control *"Babylon, which is the Mother and Producer of Prostitutes, Drug Addicts, Drunkards, Gluttons, Sodomites, Soothsayers, Kidnappers, Thieves, Liars, Rapists, Murderers, and whatever shall be Found OUTSIDE of that Holy City, called the NEW JERUSALEM!"* — just to Paraphrase it in Plain English for whomever might have an Inkling of Good Understanding concerning Worldly Affairs!

D-[ ] Fourthly, and with a Word of WARNING, **"The Great World TEMPLE of PEACE"** will Control ALL Communication Systems, Worldwide: beCause the Masses of People will VOTE for it, after we Hold: **"The Great Worldwide TELEVISED Court HEARING!" (That Great Meeting of the Most Intelligent Minds!) By The Worldwide People's Revolution!®** Book 041. Yes, we Tax Slaves, Interest Slaves, Insurance Slaves, Drug Slaves, Childcare Slaves, and Work Slaves have had ENOUGH of this MADNESS that is called "freedom of speech," which Allows almost everything to be Published, EXCEPT the Truths that are Taught by **The Worldwide People's Revolution!®**, which is Suppressed by those Lying Red JEWS, who Control the Major Publishing Companies, the News Media, the Weapons Manufacturing, and the War Games, who also Orchestrated the Evil Events of September 11th, 2001, among other Evil Events, which will be Proven at that Great Meeting of the Most Intelligent Minds, beginning with *"Experts Speak Out,"* which you can find on YouTube Videos, or at: www.AE911TRUTH.org, which Presents Irrefutable FACTS that no Honest Righteous Person can Rightly Deny! However, if you Vainly Imagine that you can Prove such "Facts" to be WRong, you are Welcome to Present your Evidences to: **"FREEDUM uv SPEECH!" (U Speshoul Maguzeen uv Onist Upinyunz!) By The Worldwide People's Revolution!®** Book 030-0002. Yes, everyone and anyone is Welcome to Present their Honest Opinions about ANY and ALL Important Subjects, which Opinions will be Graded for their Values, and Posted within that Good Magazine, FREE of Charge for everyone to Study — that is, IF we get **"The New RIGHTEOUS One-World Government"** Established BEFORE those Lying Red Jews bring about a Great Atomic NIGHTMARE! After all, they do not Care how many Innocent People that they Murder, just so long as they Escape: beCause they are Psychopaths without any EMPATHY! Yes, former President George Warmonger Bush and Little Dick Chicanery, Incorporated, are Perfect Examples of what we Mean by PSYCHOPATHS without any EMPATHY, who went to War in Afghanistan and Iraq without any Justifiable Causes: beCause America was NOT Attacked by the People of IRAQ, nor by the People of Afghanistan, who Paid the Price with MILLIONS of Lives Lost, Wounded and Displaced, which also Caused many other Disasters in the Middle East, and brought about MILLIONS of Needless Refugees! {See www.Amazon.com for: **"AIIRMWVC!" (Aliens, Illegal Immigrants, Refugees, Migrant Workers and other Victims of Capitalism!) By The Worldwide People's Revolution!®** Book 032.}

E-[ ] Fifthly, **"The Great World TEMPLE of PEACE"** will Invite Honest Intelligent Righteous People from around the World to Speak from the Throne Room of that Great Temple, which will be Interpreted into all Major Languages, and Published all around the World, whereby everyone can Hear what the RIGHTEOUS People have to Say, who have also Filled Out and Filed **"The Complete SURVEYS of our VALUES"** on the Internet for everyone to Study, whereby we might Discover their Values, and WHY they Believe whatever they Believe. The WHOLE Truths about all Important Subjects will not be Discovered, until we Hold those Great Meetings of the Most Intelligent Minds, whatever those Truths might be, which is what True Freedom of Speech is all about with a Capital T, F and S. Therefore, if you have something very Important to Say, now is the Time to get it Written down, Correctly: so that you or someone else may Present those Truths at some Great Meeting of the Most Intelligent Minds, which Speech or Sermon must be Studied by the Elected Officials of **"The New RIGHTEOUS One-World Government"** before it is Presented: so that it might be Corrected and Graded for its Values, whereby the Better Speeches will Receive Higher Priorities, which will be Played 3 Times per Day on all TV Networks, Worldwide, which will have ZERO Commercial Advertisements, and ZERO Nonsense: beCause we are talking about making almost everyone in the World Moderately RICH! {See the above Link for: **"LIGHTNING Versus the Lightning Bug!" (HOW almost Everyone can become Moderately RICH, without Telling Any Lies nor Selling Any Trash!) By The Worldwide People's Revolution!®** Book 001.}

F-[ ] Sixthly, **"The Great World TEMPLE of PEACE"** will Represent ALL Religions that Promote Goodness, Truths, and True Prosperity, even if they have some False

Doctrines, which we will Attempt to Prove to be WRong, and thus put all such False Religions to Rest with Confusionism, Communism, Socialism, Fascism, and Capitalism, among any other False Economic Systems that might Spring Up in the Thorny Briar Patch of Massive Confusion. After all, a True Economic System would not Produce Billions of Extremely Poor People, who do not even have Fresh Clean Air to Breathe, Pure Living Water to Drink, Wholesome Natural Foods to Eat, Secure Fireproof Termite-proof Tornado-proof Rot-proof Rat-proof Paint-proof Hurricane-proof Earthquake-proof Hail-proof Cockroach-proof Insurance-proof Self-air-conditioned Houses, Luscious All-Mineral Organic Gardens, nor Home-craft Workshops to Work in with Well-made Tools. Indeed, a True Economic System would have Eternal Employment for EVERYONE, even after they are all Living in **"Beautiful Swanky PALACES!" (A New Concept in Living Habits — Swanky Palaces for Poor People!) By The Worldwide People's Revolution!®** Book 066. Yes, it is all Physically and Financially Possible, O Lady Doubtfulness! Therefore, do not Cast Up any Ugly Thick Brick Walls of Unbelief in our Faces, just beCause of your Lack of Faith Hope Trust Love Patience Persistence and Obedience! {See www.Amazon.com for: **"The Seven Basic Spiritual Building Blocks of LIFE!"** Book 036, plus: **"Seven Great Armies of Working Soldiers!" (HOW to Provide a Way for Everyone to WORK: so as to Eliminate Poverty, Crimes, Drug Abuses, Prisons and Unnecessary Taxes!) By The Worldwide People's Revolution!®,** Book 015, which is a Companion Book of: **"Are you a Jobless Graduate of the SKQL uv FQLZ?" (HOW to get a GOUD EJUKAASHUN without Robbing the Bank!)**, Book 020, which is a Companion Book of: **"The Public School of IGNERUNT FQLZ!" (HOW we have been GRAATLEE DISEEVD!)**, Book 024, which is a Companion Book of all of the Books that are Listed in Chapter 20!}

00-05 [_] O Doctor Edison, it Sounds like a Capitalist Sales Pitch to me, whereby you and **The Worldwide People's Revolution!®** are Attempting to SELL a whole Bunch of Books!

00-06 [_] Well, that is True — we are most Certainly ATTEMPTING to Sell a few Billion Books, while making a few Million Wise People much Richer; but, not for any Personal Gain on our Parts. After all, our Elected King is already a Rich Person, who is not in any Great Need of Obtaining TRILLIONS of Dollars, even though that would be Helpful, if he were Burdened with the Expenses of Building those **"GLORIOUS Swanky Hotels Castles and Fortresses,"** which might be as much as 100 Miles in Diameter, and contain 10,000 **"Beautiful Swanky PALACES!"** with Millions of Stone Dome Home Complexes. However, you might be Wondering just HOW we could Afford it? Well, you should study: **"SWANGKEENOMIKS Rules the Roost!" (HOW all People can Prosper in a RIIT WAA, and STOP Polluting the Earth with Capitalist TRASH!) By The Worldwide People's Revolution!®** Book 039.

00-07 [_] O Doctor Samuel Walker Edison, I Want to Learn **"The Proper RULES for FASTING,"** which seems to be Irrelevant with those other Subjects, even as Important as they might be. Therefore, why do you not let your Elected King get on with his Inspired Book?

00-08 [_] Well, without the Construction of those **"GLORIOUS Swanky Hotels Castles and Fortresses,"** it is Doubtful that anyone will do much Fasting: beCause of the FOUL AIR, PUTRID Water, Acid Rains, Diseased Trees, Pesticides, Herbicides, Insipid Pale Fruits, and

Imitation Fruit Drinks, which are no Good for Flushing Out a Person's Bowels, after Fasting and Praying and Meditating and Doing whatever you might Do: beCause the Capitalist Environment is a Manmade DISASTER! {See www.Amazon.com for: **"The Environmentalists' Paradise!" (HOW almost Everyone could be Living in a Beautiful Manmade Paradise!) By The Worldwide People's Revolution!® Book 035.**}

00-09 [_] O Doctor Edison, I am most Thankful to God that someone is taking up **"The Swanky Sword of Divine Truths,"** whereby we might put the Devil OUT of Business, except that not one Person in a thousand Likes to READ Books, and those who do Like to read, find Romance Novels more Interesting than Fasting, who are likely to be Turned Off by all of the Capitalized Words.

00-10 [_] Well, they should Study: **"Justifications for Capitalizations!" (WHY our Elected King Defies the School of Fools by Capitalizing LOVE and HATE!)**, Book 049, which is more Understandable after Carefully Reading: **"The END of CONFUSION!" (The Great CELEBRATION of the Magnificent Wedding of the Humble Honest Nations, and the Grand Year of JUBILEE!) By The Worldwide People's Revolution!® Book 050.**

00-11 [_] O Doctor Edison, I must Humbly Confess that during all of my Life, I have never Heard such Astounding Words as you use, which has me Dumbfounded, whereby I have no Idea what to Say, except that I am DUMB-founded by DUMB-mocracy, which seems to be coming to an END! Yes, I FEAR that the Anti-Christ has Come, who is *your* Elected KING; but, NOT mine!

00-12 [_] Trust me, if the Masses of People Reject the Great Truths that are Taught by our Elected King, they will Deserve to have some Anti-Christ DICTATOR Ruling Over them: beCause that is the Price that People will Pay for Rejecting Truths without any Justifiable Causes. Indeed, one of those Great Truths is concerning the Need for People to REPENT, which Begins with FASTING and PRAYING, even as the People of Nineveh Fasted and Prayed for 40 Days and 40 Nights, according to *the Book of Jonah,* which does not even give the Sermon that was Taught by Jonah, which Jesus referred to in *Matthew 12:41,* which Clearly States: *"The Men of Nineveh shall Arise during the Day of Judgment, and shall Condemn this Wicked Generation of Evildoers: because they Repented According to the Preaching of Jonah; and behold, a Greater Prophet than Jonah is now here. Therefore, how shall you Escape the Damnation of Hell, if you Reject his Inspired Words of Provable Truths?" — The New MAGNIFIED Version (NMV) in Plain English.* Therefore, WHERE is that Sermon to be Found in your Unholy Mutilated Bible? "NOWHERE," you might say; but, that is only beCause you have not Studied *Malachi 4,* which Reveals that God will Send the Man with the Spirit of Elijah before the Second Coming of the Anointed Savior, who will Restore the Truths about all Important Subjects, including HOW to Repent. {See www.Amazon.com for: **"The Gospel According to our Elected King!" (The Good News from the Most Modern Perspective!)**, Book 013, plus: **"In thu Beeginingz uv Thingz!" (Thu Kreeaashun Stooree frum thu Beegining!)**, Book 025, plus: **"The Secret City of the Great King!" (HOW the True Church will Escape from the Great Tribulation!)**, Book 042, plus: **"The New MAGNIFIED Version of The Book of MOORMUN!" (The Story of the White and Dark Indians in the Americas!) By The Worldwide People's Revolution!®**, Book 040, which is one of the Best Books ever written, and is far better than the Original *Book of Mormon,* which is still much more Understandable than most of the *Holy Bible.*

The Menu for a Feast of Physical and Spiritual Truths!

This Book contains 10 Beautiful Photographs and 46,306 words with 213,344 characters.

— Chapter 01 —

The Objectives for Writing this Inspired Book

01-01 [_] Well, first of all, in spite of the Fact that very few People are Interested in Fasting, those who are Interested have almost nothing to Guide them in the Right Direction, and especially if they have been reading the *Scriptures,* which have ZERO Rules to Follow, in spite of having a lot to say about Fasting, itself, which I have "Quoted" in: **"HOW to Become a HOLY Man!" (40 Good Reasons WHY People Should FAST and PRAY!),** Book 045. Yes, it is one of the most Amazing Things about the *Holy Bible,* which seems to Treat or Mistreat that most Important Subject with a "Grain of Salt," as they say, which Barely Works Up an Appetite for Learning any more about it! Indeed, some People have "red" the entire Bible no less than 40 Times, and have yet to Do any Fasting: beCause of several Reasons. (Please Check any Boxes [_] with Statements that you Agree with:)

A-[_] I Agree, I have not found Time to Do any Proper Fasting: beCause of being too Busy Earning a Living. After all, I have a Family to Feed.

B-[_] I Believe that I would be Fired from my Job, if I took Time to Fast and Pray.

C-[_] I Confess that it would be Good for some People to Fast. Therefore, I will leave Fasting for the Experts — such as Jesus, Moses, and Elijah.

D-[_] The Apostle Paul Fasted often, and still Died with a Proverbial Thorn in his Side.

E-[_] Educated People know that Fasting is Beneficial. Therefore, if I get so Sick that I Lose my Appetite, then I will Fast and Pray. However, without the Permission of some Medical Doctor, who Writes out an Excuse for me, my Boss will likely Fire me from my Job with Jobe.

F-[_] I Fail to Understand WHY that I should Fast. We have Drugs that Cure almost all Common Ailments; and therefore, there is no Need for me to Fast nor Pray. Besides that, I do not Believe in Fasting: because these are Modern Times. Indeed, no Body can Heal itself without the Aid of MediSINZ. †§‡

G-[_] God knows that Fasting is for Spiritual Weaklings, like Moses and Elijah, who would not be Able to do it, nowadays: beCause of the Pollutions of Air, Water, and Land. Therefore, it is a Lost Cause. Just Forget it. Yes, Set your Mind on Good Things — such as Buying New Cars, which are Holy Things. Yes, God Knows that they are Holy! †§‡§§

H-[_] HUMBUG! Fasting is Nature's ONE and ONLY Sure Cure for all Wild and Domesticated Animals, including People, whose Bodies will more Rapidly Heal while Fasting, which can be Proven in a Courtroom with Law and Order, if you People are not Spiritual COWARDS of the Lowest Order of Lying Hypocrites!

I-[_] I am an Innocent Lamb of God, who should not have to Do any Fasting: beCause I have been Eating nothing but Wholesome Natural Foods — such as Drinking Cow's Milk, Eating Cheeseburgers, Pizzas, and Iced-creams with a thousand Added Chemicals and Poisons, plus all Kinds of French-fried Chips with Dips, which have hundreds of Preservatives and Additives, which the Baby Jesus also Ate for his Good Health; and I am NOT Insane, nor telling any Lies! †§‡§§

J-[_] Justice Demands that Ignorant People like you should be brought into a Courtroom, and Forced to Prove your Innocence: beCause you are Obviously Insane; or else you are being very Sarcastic (§), which is Permissible in this "Courtroom": because it is an Open Forum for everyone who Believes in Freedom of Speech with Justice for all.

K-[_] King Jesus would FORCE everyone in the World to Do some Fasting, even if he had to Lock them up in Prisons, just to Learn some of the Benefits for Fasting, which all Wild Animals do Naturally for Maintaining Good Health. Yes, even Domesticated Dogs and Cats often undertake Fasting, if they have Lost their Appetites to Eat. Therefore, it is a GOOD Thing to Learn all about it, and long before some Great Famine comes, when it will be Extremely Difficult to do any Fasting: beCause of a LACK of Fresh Fruit Juices.†

L-[_] Lots of Laughs! King Jesus will never be Elected to Govern **"The New RIGHTEOUS One-World Government!"** Besides that, if he had any Sense at all, he would Refuse to have anything to do with such Insane People, who cannot even Understand that the Human Body has a Way of Storing Up Buckets of Lard and Excess FILTH and Accumulated Poisons, which can only be Eliminated by Fasting. †§‡§§

M-[_] Sufficient MONEY will Solve all of our Problems, and can therefore BUY Good Health, which was Proven by Howard Hughes, who Spent Billions of Dollars on his own Good Health, and still Died with Insanity! And I Believe that I am NOT Crazy. †§‡§§

N-[_] You are a NUT — Money is a Tool of the Devil, an Invention of Satan, who is also the Chief Promoter of Drugs, which all of the Wild Animals Live Happily without. Yes, just Name ONE Drug that was Used by the Millions of American Bisons, who used to Roam on the Great Plains, who had no Hospitals, no Medical Doctors, no Drugs, nor any Use for any such Vain Things! ‡

O-[_] Are there no Options? Must we all Learn HOW to Fast and Pray, and thus Follow some Proper RULES for FASTING? Why not just Eat LESS Foods, and Natural Wholesome Foods and Drinks when we do Eat?

P-[_] People have been Eating Natural Wholesome Foods for thousands of Years, and they still had a certain Amount of Ailments: beCause of the Accumulated FILTH within their Bodies: beCause of Failing to Do some FASTING, whereby their Bodies might have had a Chance to Eliminate any Excess Filth: beCause of SHRINKING DOWN and SQUEEZING OUT those Poisons, which can be Greatly Assisted by Drinking Sweet Fruit Juices, which are otherwise called *"the Water of Life,"* in *Biblical* Terms. Yes, the Fruit Trees are the Life of Mankind, just as Moses wrote in *the Book of Deuteronomy.*

Q-[_] The Great Question is this: **"Must we Follow certain RULES for Fasting, in Order to be Successful at it?"** And the Answer is, YES: beCause thousands of Ignorant People have Fasted; but, only a Select FEW have been Successful — such as Moses and Elijah, who had the POWERS of the GODS! Therefore, the Rules must make a Great Deal of Difference.

R-[_] I will be Contented to wait around for my Resurrection from the Dead, after which Time I will be Judged for my Good Works and my Righteous Words. Meanwhile, I am going to Eat, Drink, and be Merry — just like the Rich Man in *Luke 16.* †§‡§§

S-[_] Satan has all of you Ignorant People Greatly Deceived by your Accumulated FALSE Riches, whereby you Vainly Imagine yourselves to be Rich, and have need for nothing, in spite of being Spiritually Blind, Naked, and Extremely POOR, whereby you do not even have Fresh Clean Air to Breathe, Pure Living Water to Drink, Wholesome Natural Foods to Eat, nor Secure Houses to Live in, which are Fireproof, Mouse-proof, Hail-proof, Rot-proof, Paint-proof, Termite-proof, Tornado-proof, Hurricane-proof, Self-air-conditioned, Insurance-proof and Tax-proof! Indeed, you are nothing but SLAVES — as in Work Slaves, Tax Slaves, Interest Slaves, Insurance Slaves, Drug Slaves, Sex Slaves, Childcare Slaves, and Seduced Slaves of the EVIL Empire, who are too Proud to even Confess it: beCause of your FALSE Riches, which have Blinded your Minds from the Realities of Life, whereby Satan is Bound to Drag you Down into Hell with himself, along with all of your Ignorant Children, who shall also Waste their Lives in SLAVERY!

T-[_] It is now High Time for a Worldwide REVOLUTION, whereby all of the Slaves can be LIBERATED by **"The Swanky Sword of Divine Truths!"** Book 067.

U-[_] I Understand what you People are saying; but, I am Unable to Do any Fasting: beCause I have BILLS that must be Paid! Yes, I Freely Confess that I have been Trapped in Satan's Snares, which were Set Up by the Evil Empire, which did not Teach to us Children anything about Good Health, except to not Smoke those Stinking Cigarettes, which are still found for Sale throughout the World: beCause Nicotine is the Most Addictive Drug there is, which those Lying Red Jews have known all along; and yet it is still LEGAL: beCause **"The Divided States of United Lies"** is Totally Controlled by those Lying Zionist Red Jews, who are of the Synagogue of SATAN, just as the *Holy Bible* Teaches. See *the Book of Revelation* for the Proof; and Remember that they were the Enemies of Christ, who was an Honest White Jew, who Orchestrated his Death. Yes, you can read it in *the Gospel of John* and in *the Book of the Acts of the Apostles.*

V-[_] I am Determined to get the Victory over Satan and his Evil Synagogue of Red Jew Liars, who Refuse to DEMAND: **"The Great Worldwide TELEVISED Court HEARING,"** whereby all such Important Things might be Proven in a Courtroom, and Published on all TV Channels in all Major Languages, Worldwide, all at the same Time, while all other Nonsense is SHUT OFF.

W-[_] Those Lying Zionist Red Jews would have us Tax Slaves get ourselves into another Hateful World WAR, before they would Humbly Submit to **"The Swanky**

Sword of Divine Truths!" After all, they have already Profited by TRILLIONS of Dollars from those Hateful Wars: beCause they Loan Money at High Interest Rates to Naïve Government Officials, who are not even Aware of their Scams, who have never Studied any Anti-Semitic Literature: beCause they are in LOVE with the Synagogue of Satan, even as they are in Love with their Addictive Drugs. For Example, the Taliban in Afghanistan had almost Wiped Out the Poppy Plants, which are used for making Heroine and Opium Products; but, along came the False Flag Evil Events of September 11th, 2001, which called for a WAR on Afghanistan, which Liberated those Poor People from the Wicked, WICKED Taliban, whereby they now Produce 10 Times more Poppies than ever! Yes, Heroin is now Cheaper in **"The Divided States of United Lies"** than it ever was — Thanks to American Tax Slaves, who Financed the Wars in the Middle East, at a Cost of no less than 6 Trillion Dollars! Yes, only 2 Trillion went into the Pockets of Red Jew Bankers, while the other 4 Trillion went into the Pockets of Red Jew Weapons Manufacturers, Gas Companies, Oil Industries and their Red Jew Cousins, all of whom LOVE those Hateful Wars: beCause of Greatly Profiting from them, at Tax Slaves' Expense! Yes, even the Coffin Makers, Flower Shops, Liquor Stores, and Beer Parlors Profited from them: beCause American Wars are BIG Business, and especially for Red Jew Hospitals, Medical Doctors, and Drug Manufacturers, who Rake in hundreds of Billions of Dollars! Therefore, just Follow the Money Trail, and you will Discover that it Leads straight into the Pockets and Bank Accounts of ZIONIST JEWS and their Friends. For Example, Little Dick Chicanery gained some 50 Billion Dollars by the Wars in the Middle East, which should Disturb all Righteous Honest People; but, NOT George Warmonger Bush, Incorporated: beCause they also Gained BILLIONS of Dollars! ‡

X-[_] X-amount of People are likely to HATE YOU, O Elected King, just for Publishing such Inflammatory Literature as this, which is Anti-Semitic, and therefore Anti-Christ. †§

Y-[_] I am Yearning for the Day of Justice, when the Real Criminals and Chief Criminals are put on Trial — be they White Jews or Red Jews, be they Black Jews or Brown Jews, be they Yellow Jews or Blue Jews — beCause this Capitalist MADNESS has gone on Long Enough! Yes, Babylon must FALL, and we Honest White Jews must do our Best to Help it to Fall: beCause the whole Earth is now in Danger of becoming another Desolate Planet, like Mars! Therefore, you should also be Yearning for: **"The Great Worldwide TELEVISED Court HEARING!" (That Great Meeting of the Most Intelligent Minds!) By The Worldwide People's Revolution!®** Book 041.

Z-[_] The Great ZEAL of all True Believers will make that Possible.

01-02 [_] In Fact, if there is a more Important Subject within the *Bible,* I would like to Learn what it might be, since it is Impossible to be "Saved" in any Spiritual Way without Repentance, which Begins with a Full Confession that we have done WRong in some Way, which is Usually a Wrongdoing with our DIETS, as was the Case for the People of Nineveh, who were Commanded by their King to put on Sackcloth, and Sit in Ashes, and BEG God to Forgive them, while they Fasted for 40 Days and 40 Consecutive Nights, and supposedly without Eating nor Drinking anything, which many People would call a Jewish Fairy Tale — except that none of them have any Idea just Exactly HOW the People of Nineveh did their Fasting, which is

Revealed in: **"The Gospel According to our Elected King,"** which gives the entire Sermon of Jonah, plus several other Conversations and Enlightening Bits of Information that no Seeker of Truths should be Deprived of.

01-03 [_] O Elected King, are you Actually the Man with the Spirit of Elijah? Have you come to Torment us with your Religious Doctrines, and even Set Up yourself over all of the Nations as the KING of Kings, even the Great so-called "TYRANT King" of **"The New RIGHTEOUS One-World Government,"** which will get the Household of Israel in Order, before the Second Coming of Jesus Christ?

01-04 [_] Well, it was for that Reason that I was Born, which I have no Real Interest in for any Personal Gain nor Glory; but, for your Sake, and for the Sakes of Billions of Ignorant People, someone must get Control of this Insane World, before we Destroy ourselves with some Great Atomic NIGHTMARE. After all, there are presently some Billion-plus Muslims in this World of Woes, who could be Ignited and United Against **"The Divided States of United Lies,"** and for Justifiable Causes — such as the Lying Red Jew FALSE FLAG Operations of September 11th, 2001, whereby MILLIONS of People DIED as a Result of it, or otherwise have been Wounded or Displaced by it, which can only Rightly be Settled in a Courtroom, which I have Identified as: **"The Great Worldwide TELEVISED Court HEARING!" (That Great Meeting of the Most Intelligent Minds!) By The Worldwide People's Revolution!® Book 041.**

01-05 [_] Yes, Exciting Times are Coming, O Lady Doubtfulness, when True Justice will be Served in one Way or another, and Hopefully in a very Peaceful Civilized Way, which is within a COURTROOM, where Law and Order Prevail with a Righteous Judge in Charge of it, which is MYSELF, since I am the ONE and ONLY Person on this Earth who has Reasonable and Provable SOLUTIONS for our Massive Problems! Yes, I Challenge anyone else to Present any Solutions that are Better than my own, which were Revealed to me by the Most High God of this Solar System, whose Name is YOHOOVU, in Swanky "Funetik Ingglish," which has ONE Way to Spell ONE Sound each Time, as Opposed to the 10 or more Ways to Spell Single Sounds in Standard English Confusion. {See the KEE TQ PROONUNSEEAASHUN in: **"LIGHTNING Versus the Lightning Bug!" (HOW almost Everyone can become Moderately RICH, without Telling Any Lies nor Selling Any Trash!) By The Worldwide People's Revolution!® Book 001.**}

01-06 [_] For Example, here are some very Familiar Words with many Ways to Spell the single Sound of "OO," as in: Sch**oo**l, r**u**le, d**o**, sh**oe**, thr**ough**, cr**ew**, fr**ui**t, S**iou**x, tw**o**, bl**ue**, l**ieu**, man**eu**ver, rh**u**barb, rh**eu**matism, rendezv**ous**, gh**ou**l, p**oo**h, and so on, which is nothing but Confusion within the Minds of Innocent Children, who Waste much of their Precious Time in **"The Public School of IGNERUNT FQLZ,"** when they could be Learning Important Truths from Good Books, such as: **"Thu Nq MAGNUFIID Verzhun uv Thu PROVERBZ uv KING SOLUMUN in Plaan Ingglish!" (The Understandable Version of the Famous Proverbs of King Solomon in Plain English!) By The Worldwide People's Revolution!®, Book 027,** which is mostly written in Swanky "Funetik Ingglish."

01-07 [_] So, O Elected King, WHY would you Choose a Book like this to Reveal all such Important Information in it, rather than Write another Inspired Book that Deals with that

Important Subject, only? For Example, it could be called: **"Our Elected King Who Speaks Out!" (It is High Time for some Sane Person to Get Control of this Insane World!) By The Worldwide People's Revolution!®** Book 070.

01-08 [_] Well, that Sounds like a very Good Title, which I should get onto Producing right away — except that I have a dozen or so other Inspired Books that need to be Finished, first. {See www.Amazon.com for: **"HOW to get Our PRIORITIES in ORDER!" (The Glories of Democracy; and, Does DEMON-ocracy have its Priorities in Order?) By The Worldwide People's Revolution!®** Book 060.}

01-09 [_] O Elected King, I have no Idea WHO might be Inspiring you to Write all such Silly Books; but, it is for Certain that it is NOT Jehovah God, who is NOT the Author of Confusion. (See *First Corinthians ... whatever.* I cannot rightly recall the Chapter and Verse.)

01-10 [_] Well, you most Certainly have a Right to have your Honest Opinions Expressed in my Inspired Books, even without Knowing ALL of the FACTS. After all, I am Wanted by the Federal Burden of Investigation (FBI), the Central Unintelligent Agencies (CIA), the Federal Emergency Mismanagement Agency (FEMA), the Good Drugs and Bad Foods Administration (FDA), the Infernal Revenue Snakes (IRS), the DEPARTment of Non-Organic Agriculture (DofA), the Fire DEPARTments, Worldwide, and many other Government DEPARTments: beCause I am Fixing to put ALL of them OUT of Business! Yes, they are Wanting me to be the First Person who is brought to Trial for Upsetting the Great False Economy, which is Founded on Red Jew LIES! †§ {See: **"The Great False Economy is now DEBUNKED!"** Book 053.}

01-11 [_] O Elected King, it seems that you are Prejudiced against those JEWS. So, are you Anti-Semitic, or what?

01-12 [_] Well, there are Basically 2 Kings of Jews, which are those Lying Red Jews, who can easily be Identified by their Red Ears, who are like Judas Iscariot and Bernie Madoff; and those Honest White Jews, who are like Jesus Christ and his Honest Trustworthy Disciples, who were put to Death by those Lying Red Jews called Scribes and Pharisees, who Orchestrated their Deaths: beCause their Beliefs and Doctrines THREATENED those Lying Red Jews, even as my Beliefs and Doctrines Threaten the Great EVIL Empire, which I call: **"The Divided States of United Lies!"** — which is Based in the District of Chief Criminals, in Washington and on Wall Street, in New Yuck City, where they Practice Banker-craft, who have Invented thousands of Strange Definitions for Common Words, which few People can Understand, and even fewer People have any Desire to Understand such Definitions, which are Fashioned somewhat like Medical Words, which are in Latin for the Sake of Confusion. After all, how many People Want to Bother themselves with Memorizing all such Words and their Meanings, when they only Want to LIVE? — that is, they Want to Live Healthy Happy Lives, at HOME with their Families and Friends: beCause they have no Real Interest in making Tax Slaves, Interest Slaves, Insurance Slaves, Drug Slaves, Childcare Slaves, nor Work Slaves of themselves. However, in the Process of Trying to Earn an Honest Living, they have been Sucked Into that Proverbial *"Bottomless Pit,"* which *the Book of Revelation* refers to, which also Identifies those Lying Red Jews as Belonging to *"the Synagogue of Satan,"* in *2:9 and 3:9,* which Verses do not go into any Details about them; but, the Remainder of the Book does somewhat Outline their EVIL Works, if you can Understand it. Indeed, most People do NOT Understand it, and therefore they do not Study it. Neither will I go into any Great "Boring Details" within this Inspired Book about it: beCause it is another Subject that must be Addressed in its own Book, which I may Address in the Book that is Mentioned in Verse 01-07. Moreover, we never Know for Sure what a Day will bring forth, nor what New Books that I will be Inspired to Write; but, you can be Sure that as Long as I Live, I will do my Best to put the Evil Empire DOWN: beCause it can Rightly be Blamed for almost ALL of the Massive Problems that we now have in this World of Woes — none of which were Needed, except to Teach to us certain Valuable Lessons, one of which is the Fact that most People were Born to be SERVANTS, and NOT Masters. {See www.Amazon.com for: **"A Sound Argument for Masters and Servants!" (WHY Everyone Needs a Good Master, and every Master Needs Good Obedient Servants!) By The Worldwide People's Revolution!®**, Book 008, which is a Companion Book of: **"GOOD NEWS for REBEL WOMEN!" (HOW almost all Wives can become Moderately RICH without Leaving their Homes! Guaranteed!)**, Book 010, which contains a very Special Chapter, which alone could "Turn the World Upside Down," if it were Printed and passed out on the Streets of these Cities of Confusion, which is Chapter 04 of that Inspired Book, which can easily be Printed on just 2 Sheets of Paper, which are 11 by 17 inches, which can also be Folded just Right for making a Letter to Mail Out to whomever you might Think Needs a Copy, which they can also Copy and Mail to whomever they Think Needs a Copy, and so, until at last the whole World is SATURATED with that simple Message, which is Profound and POWERFUL!

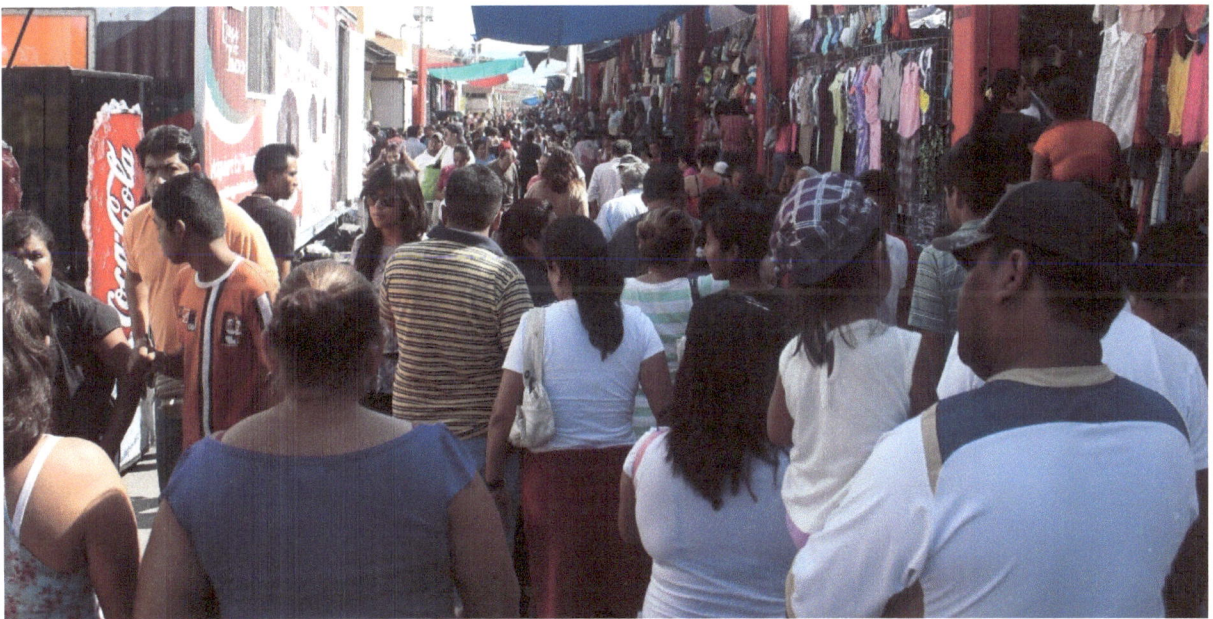

{FOOTNOTE: You can easily See that the Majority of these People are Overweight, and yet they are going Shopping for more: beCause they are not Contented with whatever they have. Therefore, this Marketplace covers nearly a Quarter of a Square Mile with Vain Things that People could Live Happily without, even as I have Lived for my entire Life without ANY of those Vain Things. Moreover, I Checked it all Out, and did not Discover even one Thing that I Wanted to Buy. Therefore, the Apostle Paul wrote, *"Be you Contented with such Things as you have in your own Garden, Vineyard and Orchard, even as Adam and Eve were Contented."*}

— Chapter 02 —

We must Understand the Human Body

02-01 [_] There are more than 5,000 Miles of Pipes — including Blood Vessels, Capillaries, the Throat, Intestines, and the Wind Pipe — within one Human Body — not Counting how many BILLIONS of CELLS that are Surrounded by POCKETS, which can Accumulate Gallons and GALLONS of EXCESS FILTH, Fat, POISONS, Oils, GREASE, and Harmful Residues, Acids, Chemicals, and Poisons, which can be Retained within the Body for 60 Years, or more: beCause that is the Way that the Human Body was DESIGNED by the Great Creator God, whose ONE and ONLY Natural Remedy is FASTING and PRAYING.

02-02 [_] Indeed, HOW ELSE could such Great Quantities of FILTH and POISONS be Thoroughly REMOVED, except by Fasting and Praying, combined with WEEPING and MOURNING, which VIBRATES the entire Body, and LOOSENS UP some of that Excess FILTH and SLIME? For Example, when a Person Stops Eating, his or her Entire Body begins to SHRINK DOWN and SQUEEZE OUT those Accumulated Poisons, Grease, Oil, Slime, Mucus, and whatever it has Collected by Means of Eating and EATING. However, most People do not Stop Eating *Long Enough* for ALL of the Internal Filth to be *Thoroughly* Removed; but, just as soon as they Supposedly get "Hungry," they EAT again, even if it is only a Bad Habit of Eating beCause of the CLOCK, and not beCause of Actually having an Appetite to Eat.

02-03 [_] Therefore, they do not Experience what it is like to be FREE from all of that Internal Filth, even as they were Free when they were little Children. However, some of them Remember the "Good Old Days," when they could RUN and PLAY all Day, and Felt Good just to be Alive! Indeed, many of them are now Suffering with Various Kinds of Aches and Pains: beCause of the Poisons that have Accumulated or Collected within their Bodies, which Poisons have not been Thoroughly Removed within 10, 20, 40, or even 80 Years, or more!

02-04 [_] However, whenever a Person gets Sick, and Vomits, or gets the Diarrhea, his Body ELIMINATES or THROWS OFF X-amount of Filth and Poisons, which Saves that Person's Life! In Fact, if People did not get Sick and Vomit, for Example, they would not Live nearly so Long as they do, which Explains WHY that some People, who seem to be Sick all of the Time, can OUTLIVE those People who seem to "never get Sick."

02-05 [_] For Example, one of my Grandfathers "never had a Sick Day during his Life," according to his Wife; but, she was Sick or in Pain most of the Time, which Caused her to do a lot of Fasting: because she just Naturally Lost her Appetite, which Caused her to Outlive her Husband by many Years: beCause his Body did not Eliminate the Accumulated Poisons and Filth that KILLED him! Moreover, the Truth is that he was also in Pain for many Years; but, he would not Confess it and would not Listen to his own Body, which was Trying to Teach a few Things to him — one of which was to STOP EATING.

02-06 [_] However, his Loving Wife would tell him that if he did not Eat, he would get Weak, which, of course, was True; but, it was not the WHOLE Truth, and nothing but the Whole Truth. In Fact, if he had Fasted, or simply Stopped Eating, until ALL of his Pains DISAPPEARED, he might have easily Outlived her by 40 Years, or more: because a Man is just Naturally Stronger and Tougher than a Wombman, even as you can Discover in the History Books. Yes, see *Genesis* in any *Bible,* and Understand that most of the Patriarchs Outlived their Wives by Decades: beCause that is an Advantage that a Man has over a Wombman: beCause of his Hard Work, which Assists his Body to Eliminate Poisons by SQUEEZING his Muscles TIGHT, for Example, while Lifting Heavy Objects — that is, IF he does not Kill himself by Overworking!

02-07 [_] Nevertheless, my Grandfather would have had to have been HUMBLE Enough to Confess the TRUE State of his HEALTH Affairs, or his INTERNAL Bodily CONDITION. But, how could he Confess his State of Filthiness, after being Taught that "Men do not Cry," "Big Boys can take the Pain, and Smile," "True Men do not Show their Feelings," and all other such NONSENSE, which Jesus Christ just Ignored? Yes, ALL of the Holy Prophets just Ignored all such Nonsense. *"Even also now, says the Supreme Ruler, Turn you to me with your Whole Heart, with Fasting, with Mourning, with Weeping and Wailing ..."* says the Holy Spirit: beCause it is GOOD for us to do so. The Truth is, **"PRIDE Comes Parading itself along in front of Destruction, and a Haughty Spirit Comes Prancing itself along in front of a Fall,"** as King Solomon WARNED.

02-08 [_] Indeed, it was PRIDE that Prevented my Grandfather from Confessing his DIETARY SINS. However, FASTING, itself and alone, will Humble a Man Sufficiently to make all such Confessions, even until he is Willing to Confess ALL Sins, including the Great SIN of Polluting the Earth with Abominations — such as those Stinking Filthy GREASY Noisy Polluting Automobiles, which were never Needed for True Prosperity: beCause it is a hundred Times more Practical to use Electric ELEVATORS and Subway TRAINS, which are a thousand Times more Efficient; but, only IF we Follow **"The Right Design for Living!" (A List of Great Advantages for Building Beautiful Planned City States!) By The Worldwide People's Revolution!®**, Book 012, which also Requires a little Humiliation and HONESTY. After all, what Big Brave PROUD American would Want to GIVE UP his Stinking Polluting Car, Pickup, Van, Truck, Bus, Tractor, Lawnmower, Snow Blower, Chainsaw, Snowmobile, Garden Tiller, Hedge Trimmer, Leaf Blower, Motorcycle, Motor Scooter, Motorboat, or any other Stinking NOISY Capitalist TRASH, while Living in **"Beautiful Swanky PALACES!"** — and in Exchange for only an Average of 4 Hours of Common Labor per Day? YES, I am talking about Palaces with Polished Marble Walls, Polished Granite Floors, Agate Windows, Waterfalls, Rivers of Living Water, HUGE Cisterns for Water Storage, Luscious All-Mineral Organic Gardens, and ZERO Bills to Pay: beCause of the DESIGNS of those Beautiful Palaces, which are Designed to Eliminate Red Jew Banksters and other Capitalist Gangsters: beCause their "services" are not Needed nor Wanted, as Saint Francis of Assisi might say!

02-09 [_] King David wrote, *"I Humbled my Soul by Means of Fasting ..."* — *Psalm 35:13, Revised King James Version (RKJV),* which you can Prove to be very Effective, just by Doing it. Therefore, if we are Truly Brave Men, we can also Humble our Souls by Means of Fasting, which is a really GOOD Idea for those of us who are not HOLY, or otherwise CLEAN in Mind, Body, and Spirit — which is what makes up a SOUL. Indeed, you are a Soul, and I am also a

SOUL; and *"The Soul that Sins shall Die"*: beCause *"the Wages of Sins are Sicknesses, Diseases, and Deaths."* — The New MAGNIFIED Version (NMV), which is Far Superior to all other Versions: beCause it is Understandable.

02-10 [_] In other Words, the Spirit will be Separated from the Body; and therefore, that Soul will be DEAD. However, according to my Beliefs, the Spirit is ETERNAL: beCause it was Created in the Image of the Invisible God, who is a Great Spirit Being, who Created all of those Spirits in the Beginning, perhaps Billions of Years Ago. {See www.Amazon.com for: **"In thu Beeginingz uv Thingz!" (Thu Kreeaashun Stooree frum thu Beegining!) By The Worldwide People's Revolution!®**, which is an Amazing Book, which is Full of New Nolij and Profound Truths, which goes back to the Creation of the Great Trionusphere, which Contains BILLIONS of so-called "Universes" like the one that we are somewhat Familiar with — except that we do not know one-trillionth of one-billionth of all that goes on in this little Universe, let alone the Great Universes, which might be a thousand Times as LARGE! Selah.}

02-11 [_] Nevertheless, even the Spirit can Die a Spiritual Death, and thus a Person can become DEAD in his Understanding, being without Good Understanding, being Unaware of Reality, being somewhat like certain Medical Doctors, who are Spiritually DEAF, who cannot Relate with the Provable Truths within this Exceptionally Good Book, nor within this Extremely Good Chapter, much less the Great Truths within: **"Did God or Satan Ordain Medical Doctors??" (Ask Huck Finn and/or Nigger Jim: because neither Tom Sawyer nor Judge Thatcher would Know!) By The Worldwide People's Revolution!®** Book 022. Moreover, they can also become LIARS and Murderers, such as those Scribes and Pharisees, who Orchestrated the Murder of the Best Person who ever Lived: beCause they Hated their Brother without a Just Cause, even as many People nowadays will no doubt Hate me for putting them Out of Business, without Realizing that they would be a hundred Times Better Off to be Living in those **"Beautiful Swanky PALACES!" (A New Concept in Living Habits — Swanky Palaces for Poor People!) By The Worldwide People's Revolution!®** Book 066.

02-12 [_] Indeed, those Scribes and Pharisees could not Tolerate the TRUTHS that Jesus Christ Taught, and therefore they Hated him; but, not for any Good Reasons. Likewise, many People Hate ME, just for telling them that they are like Morbid Cauldrons of Bubbling SCUM: beCause they STINK from their Stinking Feets to the Crowns of their Itching Heads! Yes, it OFFENDS them; but, only beCause they are Guilty of Dietary SINS!

02-13 [_] However, none of the Innocent Children are Offended by the Truth: because they are not Full of FILTH. Likewise, whomever Humbles himself — even at the Age of 80, like Moses did, according to *Deuteronomy 9* — by Means of Fasting and Praying, until he becomes like an Innocent Child with a Purified Mind and a Clean Body, is not at all Offended: beCause he is no longer Guilty of Committing Dietary Sins. Therefore, if you are Offended by what I have Written, you should Humble your Soul by Means of Fasting: because you are Unclean. Furthermore, you should Pray for Forgiveness of all of your Dietary Sins: beCause those are probably your Worst Sins, which Cause your other Sins, which are Transgressions of God's Divine Laws. (See: **"Do Christians have to OVERCOME their Sins, and STOP Sinning, in Order to be SAVED?"**)

02-14 [_] Now, you might be Wondering WHY that a Person should PRAY, and what Connection it has with FASTING? Well, the Mind, Body, and Spirit are ONE Unit — being TOGETHER as ONE; and only Death can Separate them: because the Spirit will not just Abandon the Body for nothing: beCause it Needs a Body to Live within, whereby it too can Enjoy the Wonders of the Worlds by Means of the SENSES.

02-15 [_] However, it Appears that many Minds have Abandoned the Bodies of many Americans, who seem to be in a State of Morbidity, or Rottenness, who cannot even Concentrate on what I have to say, whose Minds are Distracted by Vain Thoughts — as if this Inspired Book were far too Boring, Unenlightening, Uninspired, or whatever. {FOOTNOTE: If you Agree with them, please Check the above Box with an X, like this: [X]. Likewise, Check any other Boxes with Statements that you Agree with, which you will find most Interesting during the next Time that you Read this Inspired Book, whereby you will be Asking yourself: "Why in the World did I Check *that* Box?"}

02-16 [_] However, the next Time that they get Sick, they will perhaps give this Subject some Serious Attention — even though it will be a little too Late, if they have Lost their Minds, and have gone Crazy, or just Senile! And do not Think that YOU cannot Lose *your* Mind: because nearly a *quarter* of Old People in **"The Divided States of United Lies"** have already Lost their Minds to some Degree, and some — being like former President Ronald Reagan — have Completely Lost their Minds! Moreover, to some Degree, even the Children seem to have Lost their Riit Miindz: beCause they have Appetites to Eat Various Kinds of Garbage Foods, or Junk Foods, while Rejecting Natural Wholesome Foods: because their Minds and Bodies are Perverted by *Repetitious Advertisements,* or by what the *Bible* Identifies as *Chants* or *ENCHANTMENTS,* and by the Junk Foods that they Buy beCause of those Enchantments. {See: **"DIETS!" (A Reasonable Solution for the "Eternal Controversy"!) By The Worldwide People's Revolution!® Book 037.**}

02-17 [_] Indeed, they CHANT the same Repetitious Advertisement, over and OVER: beCause they Know that it Works Properly to Instill LUSTS within Weak Minds, and thus it Works Well to SELL their TRASH: beCause Weak-minded People Allow such Lusts into their Minds. Therefore, that is a Major Reason WHY that they should Fast and Pray.

02-18 [_] However, most of the Children have just been Fed whatever their Parents have Imagined is Good for them, or whatever was Advertised to them by Radios, TV's, Computers, iPhones, Books, Billboards, Newspapers, or whatever. Therefore, the Children cannot be Blamed for their Mental nor Physical Weaknesses, which are the Result of a LACK of Proper Natural Minerals, Vitamins, and Enzymes (among other Things, like a Lack of Exercise, and True Love, which does not come in Bottles nor in Plastic Wrappers), which are found in Fresh Unpoisoned RAW Fruits and Vegetables, which have been Grown by: **"The LUSCIOUS All-Mineral Organic Method of Gardening!" (HOW to Grow DELICIOUS Satisfying Foods for Potential Kingz and Kweenz in Swanky PALACES!) By The Worldwide People's Revolution!®,** Book 021 which is an Ancient Natural Method, which just Naturally Occurs in Territories that are Down River from Glaciers, which Lands are Fertilized by Glacial Waters, which usually contain an Abundance of Minerals, which come from POWDERED ROCKS.

02-19 [_] Therefore, when such People, who Live within such Countries, get something to Eat, it is more Satisfying to them than those Foods that are Eaten in Countries that have De-mineralized Topsoil, or NO Topsoil, which Foods are Unsatisfying to them, even if they Stuff themselves with all such Foods, Daily. Therefore, because such People are basically Starving for those Vitamins and Minerals, they keep on Eating and EATING, while Literally Starving to DEATH!

02-20 [_] However, there is a Remedy, and that is to FAST and PRAY: beCause the Body and Mind can get itself Back into the Right Order again, IF it is given a Chance, according to **"The Proper RULES for FASTING!"**

02-21 [_] **Nevertheless, if the Body is NOT given a Chance to get itself in Order, it will REBEL, and go into a Deep Depression, or do whatever it has to Do, in Order to Control the Abuser, and to Save itself from the Offender.** In Fact, the Body has a Mind of it own, which can take Total Control of the Mind, and put a Person into a COMA, or even Cause him or her to go INSANE, becoming Uncontrollable, except by Physical Restraints, like Handcuffs and Straitjackets.

02-22 [_] Such is often the Case during Wars, wherein Soldiers just "Flip Out," as they say, and Imagine themselves to be People that they are not, such as Wyatt Earp or Jesse James. And others just sit and Stare into "Outer Space": beCause their Minds are Bewildered and Dumbfounded by what has Happened around them. Therefore, the Best Remedy for them is to FAST and PRAY: because it is the one and only Sure Cure for Mental Illnesses.

02-23 [_] Likewise, whenever any Person gets a Disease, his most Reliable Remedy is to FAST and PRAY, followed by a Natural Diet of Fresh Fruits and Unpoisoned Vegetables, which have been Grown without Harmful Chemicals and Poisons — such as the Sweet Fruits from the Tree of Life, which can only be Found in the *Garden of Eden,* which was Planted by the Holy Angel, called EDEN, which is still there in the Blest Land of Perfect Oneness, in the Paradise of Peace and True Happiness, where the little Birds of Cheerfulness are Singing, and the Fragrant Flowers are Blooming by the River of Life, or the River that Gives Life from Living Waters!

02-24 [_] However, such a Person should be Wise, and Carefully Follow **"The Proper RULES for FASTING!" (The Complete Instruction Manual for True Repentance!) By The Worldwide People's Revolution!®**, which, of course, is this Good Book, just in Case some Mentally Deprived Person has already Forgotten the Title of it, which is often the Case when someone is just Listening to a Book being "red" to them, which can Happen to anyone who is half Asleep, which is often the Case: beCause all such Pure Truths have a Tendency to put People to SLEEP, even as the *Holy Bible* does in most Cases, which Explains WHY half or more of the Church Members are Asleep before the Service is Over — that is, unless some Irreverent LOUDMOUTH Sloth-gut Windbag Hole-in-his-Head is giving some LOUD Fiery Sermon — in which Case he will Naturally be Identified as "a Good Preachers," who is a Near Relative of a "Good Politician," who also has to Fire Up his Vocal Cords with some Hot Peppers, you might say, and Spice his Speech with FEARS of Coming Wars, Higher Taxes, and so on, who almost always Promises to FIX whatever is WRong, without ever Explaining just Exactly HOW he or she Plans on Doing it, whereas, in my Case, I have Explained ALL of the Fine Details within 350+ Inspired Books, which I do not Expect very many People to Study; but, if I can just

Persuade them to Study ONE Extremely Good Book — such as: **"The New MAGNIFIED Version of The Book of MOORMUN!" (The Story of the White and Dark Indians in the Americas!)**, Book 040, I will be very Happy for it, and also Consider it to be a Great Success: beCause, not even the Best of Authors have Managed that Feast, including the Authors of the *Holy Bible,* who would be rather Disappointed to Learn that less than one Percent of the People in the World have "red" it from Cover to Cover: beCause they cannot Understand it — that is, until they "reed" the New MAGNIFIED Version of it in Plain English, beginning with **"Thu Nq MAGNUFIID Verzhun uv Thu PROVERBZ uv KING SOLUMUM in Plaan Inggglish,"** which is one of my Favorite Books, which is right next to its "Twin Brother," called: **"ECCLESIASTES UNCOVERED!" (The New MAGNIFIED Version of Ecclesiastes and the Song of Solomon in Plain English!)**, Book 034, which is much Shorter!

02-25 [_] All such Inspired Books are Provided by God for Humble Honest People who Want to get Perfectly Well without Wasting any Money on Medical Snakes, whose Heads are Filled with Poisonous Lies, who Strike at the Colorful Peacock from Angel Ridge with the Poisonous Fangs of Hate and Revenge: beCause, **"The Swanky Sword of Divine Truths"** Threatens to put them Out of Business, and Permanently so: beCause of Building those **"GLORIOUS Swanky Hotels Castles and Fortresses,"** which have more than 5,000 Advantages over Cities of Confusion!

02-26 [_] However, if you are in Love with Drugs, MediSINZ, or Medicines, Shots, Pills, Potions, Lotions, Chemical Therapies, and Poisons of Various Kinds, even as ALL of the Wild Animals have been in Love with them for thousands of Years, then ENJOY your Ailments, Doctor Bills, Hospital Bills, and Endless PILLS and BILLS, even as those Wild Animals have been Enjoying them! §§ Yes, I speak very Sarcastically: because neither they nor I have Consumed ANY of those Drugs, nor Smoked any Weeds, and I can Honestly say that I do not have a single Pain within my entire Body, even though I am a bit Grieved for the Unbelief that I am Confronted with by Ignorant People, who are Afraid to even Experiment with my Inspired Words of Provable Truths, which they can all Prove by PRACTICING FASTING, according to my RULES, which make Fasting rather Pleasant and Enjoyable, if not Sensual and Erotic!

02-27 [_] Now, let it be Understood that ALL Drugs and Addictive Foods and Drinks are Unnatural, Unnecessary, Unwanted by Holy People, and Grossly Deceptive: beCause, even though such Drugs and "Treatments" might STOP the *Elimination* of whatever Filth is within a Body, those Drugs and "Treatments" do not Help the Body to Eliminate those Poisons; but, they simply SHOCK the Body, and Restrain it from doing what it would Naturally do by Means of Fasting and Praying, Combined with Weeping and Mourning and Confessing ALL Sins, including those "Transportation Sins," which we can call "Biological Sins," or "Environmental Sins," which most of us have Contributed to without Realizing the Sinfulness of it, much less the Heavy Price that the Earth will have to Pay for it, if we do not take some Immediate Action to REVERSE the Situation, and Cooperate with NATURE. After all, the Gas, Coal, Oil, and other Natural Resources of Energy were Designed for a "World-time" Supply for MILLIONS of Years, which we have already Wasted! Indeed, with much LESS Energy, we could have already Built MILLIONS of Beautiful Planned City States, called: **"GLORIOUS Swanky Hotels Castles and Fortresses,"** whereby we could have STOPPED Polluting the Earth. However, God Wanted us to Discover how STUPID we are! {See www.Amazon.com for: **"Are Americans the Most STUPID People who ever Lived?" (HOW Working People can PROSPER and Live**

in PEACE Under the Rulership of a RIGHTEOUS KING!) By The Worldwide People's Revolution!® Book 047.}

02-28 [_] Now, I Hear someone, who is like an Innocent Lamb, bleat: "O Colorful Peacock, I Fail to Understand just HOW that Fasting and Praying can *Heal* a Human Body, no matter what Ails it. Therefore, would you please Explain it to us." Well, O Lamb, when you STOP Eating, the Body continues to Eliminate or get Rid of whatever it does not Want, in Order to Grow and Nourish itself. Therefore, if there are any Excess Poisons or Filth within a Body, it will get slowly but surely SQUEEZED OUT while Fasting: beCause the entire Body SHRINKS DOWN while Fasting: beCause it is not being Fed or STUFFED with Foods.

02-29 [_] Therefore, when you Stop Eating, your Stomach and Intestines get smaller and smaller and smaller, along with all other Parts of your Body that have Accumulated or Collected any Excess Foods, which have been *Deposited* here and there by Means of the Bloodstream, which Filth is also *Eliminated* by the Bloodstream, which you could say is Running in Reverse while Fasting, whereby it is "Undoing" the Damage that was Done while Eating too much. Therefore, when your Body Shrinks Down, your Skin is left LOOSE and FLABBY: beCause the Fat and Water that was underneath the Skin has Disappeared by Means of the Bloodstream, which can Work both Ways — either to Deliver Fat and Water, or else to Remove it — and therefore, a Person can Look rather Skinny and Sickly while Fasting: because he or she does not Look "Fat nor Fair," as they say; but, such a Person is Actually less Apt to Die with a Heart Attack, Stroke, or whatever: beCause of getting Rid of at least SOME of the Sticky Gooey Stuff that makes those Heart Attacks and Strokes Possible, which is commonly called PLAQUE. Yes, it Builds Up within the Arteries while Eating, and gets Eliminated while Fasting, which is WHY it normally shows up on People's Tongues when they Fast, which you can Scrape Off with a Spoon, and then Smell of it, just to Notice that it is like "Bad Breath."

02-30 [_] Indeed, such a Fasting Person might even Appear to be PALE or SALLOW-Looking: beCause of that Plaque, which is Reflected on the Skin of the Face, which Reflects the Internal Condition of the Body; but, given Time, a Fasting Person will Eliminate all of that Filth, as well as any Lumps, Tumors, Abscesses, Cancers, or whatever the Body Wants to get Rid of: beCause it is Able and Willing to REGENERATE itself, even as Elihu Explained to Jobe in Chapter 33, which I have Greatly Magnified in some other Book for your Enlightenment. (I cannot Honestly Remember just Exactly which Book it is found in; but, I Guarantee it to be there, somewhere. Moreover, being a "one-man army," as they say, I have not yet gotten around to making a Master Index of all of the Books.)

02-31 [_] Therefore, a Fasting Person can Feel as Healthy as he has ever Felt during his entire Life, while being nothing more than "Skin and Bones," so to speak: because he is Relieved of so much Internal Filth and Poisons, which Caused him to Feel Bad while he was Eating. Indeed, it is somewhat like getting the Diarrhea — which is a Radical Elimination of Excess Poisons and Filth through the Rectum and Anus — which, when Fully Eliminated, makes a Person Feel Clean Inside, which can also Cause some Sensitive People to not Want to Eat anything: beCause they Feel so GOOD after Eliminating so much Filth and so many Poisons, which would otherwise Poison the entire Body, and could Cause Tumors in the Liver, if it were not Eliminated by the Diarrhea, Vomiting, Sweating, or by some other Means — such as Oozing Out of an Open

Sore on the Leg, which often Happens to Soldiers during Wars in Jungles, which is called "Jungle Rot," which, like Pimples and Boils, will just Disappear after Fasting on nothing but Pure Water for 2 to 3 Weeks.

02-32 [_] In Fact, even the Common Cold is just an Elimination of Excess Mucus and Slime that has Accumulated within the Human Body. Therefore, once it is Eliminated, that Person Feels much Better than before it was Eliminated — even though many People Feel WEAK: because they do not know HOW to Assist their Bodies, in Order to THOROUGHLY Clean OUT their Body Systems by Feasting on Fresh Raw Ripe Fruits, which are very Laxative — such as Fresh Figs, Peaches, Apricots, Pears, Apples, Plums, and especially Prunes, which are Dried Plums, which might not be very Fresh; but, they are very Laxative. In other Words, they will go through your Bowels quite Rapidly, as if a little Army of House Cleaners went Marching through your Bowels with Brooms and Brushes in Hand — that is, IF those Plums were Grown by **"The LUSCIOUS All-Mineral Organic Method of Gardening!"** Book 021.

02-33 [_] However, if you are STARVED for Foods, you will have to Eat a LOT of those Fruits, in order for the Body to Reject them, or Eliminate them, at which Time the Bowels will be SWEPT OUT by the Roughage of the Fruits, taking along with it as much Excess Slime and Mucus as is Possible, which is the very Slime and Filth that has been Tormenting you, all along, which could put you into Bad Moods. For Example, Refined White Sugar in Cokes, Cakes, Candies, Cookies, Pies, Iced-creams, and all such "Goodies," can Rightly be Blamed for Causing Headaches, and especially Migraine Headaches, which will simply Disappear after a few Days of Fasting, followed by a Pure Fruit Juice FLUSH — such as Fresh Squeezed Orange Juice, and a whole Gallon of it during 2 Hours or less, after going Dry for the previous 2 Days, after Drinking only Pure Spring Water previous to that, which will be Difficult to Do, if you have a Severe Headache, which could be Immediately Relieved in some Cases by taking an Enema, which will be Explained later on. The Main Thing is to Remember to NOT Eat any more White Sugar after you Recover from it: because that will Invite the "Enemy" to Return with more Vigor than ever! {FOOTNOTE: A single small Coke has as much as 10 Teaspoons of Sugar in it.}

02-34 [_] Now, you might be wondering WHERE all of that Slime and Filth might be Coming From, Originally, when you "Catch" the Cold? Well, it comes from Various Kinds of Foods, which Produce STICKY Slime within the Body, which can be Difficult to Blow OUT of your Nose, or Cough Out of your Throat, or Pass Out of your Bowels, which is referred to by Medical Doctors as a Case of "Constipation," if your Bowels will not "Move." However, the entire Body can become somewhat Constipated with all such Sticky Slime.

02-35 [_] For Example, if you have ever Eaten a Piece of Chicken with your Bare Fingers, you have no doubt Noticed that some of it STUCK to your Fingers: beCause it is like GLUE to some Degree, which comes in Different Degrees of Stickiness, depending on HOW the Chickens were Raised, and what they were Fed, which are Especially "Good Tasting" when they are Raised Properly, by **"The LUSCIOUS All-Mineral Organic Method of Gardening!"** In Fact, those Fried Chickens can be at least 10 Times "Better" than those Commercially-grown Agribusiness Abominations, which not even a Respectable Dog would Eat, after being Spoiled by some "Real" Fried Chicken at a Royal Swanky Buffet! Nevertheless, when that Super-sticky Slime gets Lodged within your Pipe Systems, it can be most Difficult to Remove by Means of a

"Common Cold," which might Require the Body to call for HELP by Means of a FEVER, which the Body is Willing to Do for the Victim of Capitalism, who cannot Distinguish one Chicken from another, which, itself, is another Great Deception: beCause the Chicken that is Grown Properly is much more Satisfying, whereby just one Leg or one Wing of it might Satisfy your Hunger for those Necessary Proteins, as Opposed to a whole Bucket of Kentucky Fried Lies!

02-36 [_] Likewise, all Kinds of Flesh produce BROTHS when they are Boiled, which People have used for thousands of Years to make SOUPS, Furniture Glues, Jellies, Jams, and whatever: beCause there are a million and one Concoctions of this and of that, according to the Inventive Imaginations of Cooks, whereby BILLIONS of Recipes have been made, and Sold in Millions of Cook Books; but, none of those Recipes can Compete with the Fine Natural Flavors of Properly-grown FRUITS — such as the 5,000+ Varieties of Mangos, the 5,000+ Varieties of Apples, the 200+ Varieties of Dates, Figs, Peaches, Pears, Plums, Apricots, Cherries, and all Kinds of Berries, which 99.999,999,999% of the People in this World of Woes have never Tasted: beCause they cannot be Found for Sale in Gross Grocery Stores! Therefore, do not Waste your Precious Time Looking for any such Fruits in such Stores, which, for the most part, are also not Found in so-called "Health Food" Stores, which Sell "Orgimmick" Produce, which does perhaps have the Advantage of not being so Poisoned; but, when it comes to Exotic and Erotic Flavors, you would have to Visit Mount Zion, and get a Basket of Good Fruits from the Garden of the Great King, himself! (See *Psalm 48, Gay King James Version {KJV}*, which is more Accurate than some of those Modern Versions, none of which Reveal the Whole Truth about anything.)

02-37 [_] Too much Meat Broth is Guaranteed to Cause the "Common Cold," as well as many other Ailments, which might Explain WHY the Wise Israelites Limited themselves to Meats on Holy Days, only, which Happened about 7 Times per Year. Some Families Adopted the "one meal of meat per week" Plan, which might have been a single Piece of Chicken, Turkey, Lamb, Kid, or whatever was handy at the Time, whereby they Avoided the RAVENOUS Appetites that many Vegetarians Obtain by Denying themselves of all Flesh, who sometimes "Sneak" into those "All-you-can-Eat" Not-so-Royal Swankless Buffets, and Gorge themselves on as many Shrimps and Tuna Salads as they can Hold, whereby they might Sweat all Night from the Heat that is Generated by all Flesh Feasts, who do not even know that Shrimps are Scavengers, who Live on DUNG, even as Farm Chickens Eat behind the Cows and Hogs, which is still quite an Improvement over the "Factory Farmed Chickens," who are Fed Growth Hormones, which Cause Children to develop Strange Breasts.

02-38 [_] Therefore, when those Sticky Foods Collect within the Bowels, they often Cause Middle-aged Men to look Pregnant: beCause it can become too Sticky to Work its Way Out of their Bowels: beCause of Stuffing themselves with such Sticky Foods, which have not been Thoroughly Eliminated for YEARS, in most Cases. Therefore, they are often Grumpy and Miserable, having ITCHES, Pains, Aches, Sores, Bleeding Hymnal-roids, and other "Top and Bottom Secret Ailments," you might say: because the Body can barely Handle it, let alone Eliminate it by Natural Means.

02-39 [_] In Fact, some People are so Stuffed with Excess Filth that their Bodies are so Weakened by it, that they cannot have a Normal Elimination through their Bowels; but, they must use **Enemas,** or Internal Water Injections through their Anuses, in Order to get Bowel

Movements at all! In other Words, they Suffer with *Chronic* Constipation of the Bowels, which often Causes Chronic Constipation of their Minds! However, all Parts of the Body can become Constipated, or Clogged Up with Sticky Filth, including the Pores of the Skin, which fill up with Grease, which then Rots and Turns BLACK, which are called Blackheads, which often develop into Pimples or Pustules that BURST OPEN on the Skin, which allows the Grease or whatever to be Eliminated by a Secondary Means, rather than be Eliminated through the Bowels. Indeed, not only are Blackheads and Pimples Eliminated through the Skin; but, Boils and Lumps are also Eliminated, which are Accumulations of Internal FILTH. Moreover, this Nolij is nothing New, as some People might Imagine; but, it is Ancient Nolij that MOSES often Mentioned within his Inspired Writings.

02-40 [_] For Example, Moses Mentioned the Common Cold in *Numbers 11,* which you can Prove to be True for yourself, just by Scientifically Experimenting with the Over-consumption or Over-eating of FLESH of any Kind — including that of Quails, Chickens, Turkeys, Ducks, Hogs, Sheeps, Goats, Cattles, Deers, Horses, Dogs, Skunks, and all Kinds of Fishes and Sea Creatures; but, Especially by Eating the Flesh of Animals that have CONCENTRATED Slimy Glue, such as Snakes and Scavengers like Vultures and Catfishes. Therefore, go ahead and be Scientific, and Experiment with Eating, if you are Brave Enough; or else Accept Moses' Words for it, and Trust your *Bible* to be True concerning that Valid Point: because it contains Ancient Provable Truths and Wisdom.

02-41 [_] Furthermore, you can Confirm what Moses wrote, by reading what King David wrote in *Psalms 78 and 103,* which are like Hidden Treasures in the Treasure Chest of the Great King. Nevertheless, even if you do not Believe anything that is written within the *Bible,* you can still Believe that certain Foods CAUSE certain Ailments: because, **for every Effect, there must be a CAUSE.**

02-42 [_] And, in most Cases, whoever Transgresses the Dietary Laws must Pay for it with certain Sicknesses and Diseases, either now or later, unless that Person Eats so little of that Food, that it becomes Meaningless — such as one Piece of Candy once during a Year, or one Piece of Chicken once per Month. Indeed, you can make yourself Sick within just ONE Day, by Overeating on one large Heavy-duty Greasy Pizza, which is enough to make a Hog Vomit — except that Hogs do not Vomit: because they know when to Obey their Loss of Appetite, and thus STOP Eating.

02-43 [_] In other Words, when they Lose their Appetites, they simply STOP Eating: because they are not Hungry; but, People are *Over-stimulated* by their LUSTS, or Longing Desires, which have been Instilled into them by Repeated Advertisements, or Enchantments, which have Caused them to WANT *more* than is Good for them.

02-44 [_] However, even *without* Advertise-Mints, some People just Naturally Think about Foods most of the Time: because they are ADDICTED to them. Therefore, their only Hope for an Escape from that Awful Deep Dark PIT, is to FAST and PRAY, According to the RULES, which is a Sure Cure; but, only IF they Confess their Lusts, and Change their Ways of Thinking. Yes, they must put the Thoughts of Eating OUT of their Minds, by Refusing to Think about any

Foods. Otherwise, they will not be Able to Fast: because they will be Overcome by the *Thoughts of Eating*, being their own Worst Enemy, you might say.

02-45 [_] However, ***"Blest are those Wise People, who Overcome their Lusts: because they shall Inherit Glory in the Holy Kingdom of All that is Good."*** (See *the Book of Revelation,* which clearly states that the *"Filthy People shall still be Filthy ..."* during the Judgment Day, if they do not Overcome their Bad Habits, including their Dietary Sins. See *Chapter 22,* and Believe what it Reveals: because it is the TRUTH. After all, would you Want to be Living in a Kingdom that was made up of Barking Dogs, Stinking Highly-Perfumed Skunks, Lying Poisonous Snakes, Vicious Lions, Greedy Hogs, and Mean Bears? I would not!)

02-46 [_] Now, that brings up another Good Reason WHY that People should Fast and Pray: beCause, after much Fasting and Praying, a Person has a Correct Sense of what is Good for him or her — that is, unless he or she Kills him or herself by Failing to Follow **"The Proper RULES for FASTING,"** in which Case he or she will not have any Senses at all.

02-47 [_] Nevertheless, ***if there is any Doubt in your Mind about the GOODNESS of Fasting, it can be Cured by simply Doing it Properly.*** However, even without doing it Properly, you can still Benefit from Fasting and Praying: because any Amount of it will usually Help to Enlighten your Mind, even if you only Fast for 24 Hours each Day, and then Eat one Moderate Meal of Fruits or Vegetables, until you Lose 10 to a hundred Pounds, if you Weigh too much.

02-48 [_] However, for those Wise People, who Want to Climb Up onto the Top of the Mountain of Good Understanding with Moses and Elijah, they will Learn HOW to Fast and Pray Properly, in Order to Obtain the GIFTS of the Supreme Ruler, who Wants to Bless them with Various Kinds of Good Gifts, including the Gift of Holiness, which is a State of Mind, Spirit, and Body wherein a Person is FILLED with the Holy Spirit, even as it was during the Day of Pentecost, when the Disciples were Gathered Together by Means of Fasting and Praying, until they were Baptized with FIRE, or SUBMERSED in Fire from God, which did not Burn them; but, it Blest them with the Gift to Speak in other Languages, which they had not Learned, among other Gifts.

02-49 [_] In other Words, they could Teach total Strangers whatever Truths came into their Minds, which Caused Multitudes of Humble People to be Converted to the Christian Religion, who also Humbled themselves by Means of Fasting and Praying, until they were also Baptized with Fire and were Filled with the Holy Spirit. Indeed, many of them did all Kinds of Miracles in the Name of Jesus Christ, who is Yoshua Messiah, the Anointed Savior, who was the Chosen Son of the Most High Ruler, who came into this World to Save those People who are Lost and Confused, who Believe in him and Obey him. Therefore, he did all Kinds of Miracles to Prove that his Words were Revealing the Truth: because he had the Fullness of the Power of God, all beCause he Loved and Obeyed the Spirit of God.

02-50 [_] See *Matthew 4,* which tells about Jesus Fasting for 40 Days in the Wilderness, where he was Tempted by Satan AFTER he became Hungry, which was after 40 Days and 40 Nights of Fasting and Praying. Likewise, the Apostle Paul did a lot of Fasting and Praying, even as all of the Saints did: because that is the Straight and Narrow Way that Leads unto Everlasting Good Health, which few People Discover. Therefore, the Apostle Paul wrote, *"Therefore, having those*

Promises, dearly Beloved — that God's Holy Spirit will Live within us, and that we will be God's Adopted Children — let us Cleanse ourselves from all Filthiness of the Flesh and Spirit, Perfecting HOLINESS in the Fear of the Supreme Ruler." (See *Second Corinthians 6 and 7,* and do not Assume that Paul was Unaware of the INTERNAL *Filthiness* of the FLESH, which comes Out of a Person when he FASTS: because Paul Assisted many People to do their Fasting, and Encouraged them to Fast: because he Knew it would Save them from their Torments. In Fact, there were more than 200 People on a Ship, whom he Persuaded to Fast and Pray: because they were in Great Peril in the Mediterranean Sea; but, after 15 Days of Fasting, they were all Saved from Destruction. See *the Book of Acts, Chapter 27.*)

02-51 [_] Likewise, the Men, Wombmen, Children, and even the Beasts of Nineveh, all Fasted for 40 Days and 40 Nights, according to *the Book of Jonah,* which Jesus called *True Repentance.* (See *Matthew 12:41.*)

02-52 [_] Likewise, Job, Abraham, Isaac, Jacob, Joseph, Samuel, David, Isaiah, Daniel, Ezekiel, Jeremiah, Amos, and many others FASTED and PRAYED for many Days: because it is the KEY that Unlocks the Door of Enlightenment, as you can Prove for yourself; but, only if you are not a Spiritual COWARD.

02-53 [_] However, because of all of the EXCESS Filth within the Bodies of most People, it is Extremely Difficult for them to Fast: because that Filth is very Ancient, Morbid, Rotten, and STINKING, which gives to them **BAD Breath,** which is another Reason that they should CONTINUE to Fast, until all of that Stink is THOROUGHLY Removed.

02-54 [_] Moreover, they might also Notice that their Tongues are Heavily COATED with a Layer of Yellowish Slime, which some People call "Plaque," which not only Covers their Tongues; but, it also Covers the Linings of their Stomachs and Arteries, as well as many other "Cells" and Internal Organs, where it is "Locked Up."

02-55 [_] However, if they are Persistent, they can Eliminate all of that Stinking Slime, and become Free from it, at which Time they will be like Holy People in their BODIES, if not also in their Spirits: because a Person Naturally Grows *Spiritually* while Fasting; but, some People Refuse to Accept the WHOLE Truth, and therefore they do not become Holy, like Moses, whose Face still Shines with the Glory of the Gods.

02-56 [_] For Example, most of the Famous Religious People throughout History either Voluntarily Fasted and Prayed, or else they were Forced to Fast and Pray, which Caused their Minds to Work like they are Supposed to, which gave to them Leadership Abilities, as well as certain Improvements in their Health. And that Explains WHY that such People as Mozart and Handel were Born: because their Parents went through a Time a Famine, just before they were Conceived; and therefore, they had very little to Eat, which was also the Case for my own Parents during World War 2, when Foods were Rationed.

02-57 [_] Likewise, such was the Case for many American Presidents, whose Parents were very Poor — such as Abraham Lincoln, "Ike" Eisenhower, and Richard Nixon, who did not always use their Intelligence Wisely; but, they still Proved that their Brains at least Worked somewhat like Brains are Supposed to, which was also the Case for Albert Einstein, Michelangelo, Leonardo da Vinci, the de´ Medici Family of Italy (the Founders of Modern Medicine), Andrew Carnegie (the Steel Magnate), John D. Rockefeller (the Oil Tycoon), and many Musicians, Artists, Actors, Actresses, Doctors, Lawyers, Teachers, Professors, Preachers, Inventors, Scientists, and so on: because Overfed People have Unclean Seeds to Sow in Filthy Unclean Wombs; but, Hungry People usually have Clean Seeds to Sow in Clean Wombs. Indeed, Jesus said that you can tell what Kinds of Trees they are by the Kinds of Fruits that they Bear: because, *"a Healthy Tree does not Bear Sick Fruits, and neither does a Sick Tree Bear Healthy Fruits. Therefore, you shall Know them by their Fruits, which are their Children."* — *NMV*. See *Matthew 7:16—20.*

02-58 [_] Therefore, that alone is another Good Reason to Fast and Pray, even if you do not Love yourself Enough to do it: because you might Love your Children Enough to do it for their Sakes. Moreover, the Apostle Paul refers to Unclean Children, who are Born from Unclean Parents, which only makes Good Sense: because all of Nature Teaches the same Great Truth. See *First Corinthians 7:14, KJV.* Indeed, Sick Animals Produce Sick Offsprings. Therefore, even if you do not Believe the *Bible,* you can still Believe what *Nature* is Trying to Teach to you: because it has no Reason to tell LIES, since Nature has nothing for Sale. However, you must be very Careful about HOW you *Interpret* what Nature is Teaching: because it too can Deceive you, if your Mind is not Working like it should, and Especially if you are Presumptuous.

02-59 [_] Now, have you ever Noticed how EM-BARE-ASSED that most People are when they enter into a Restaurant to Eat? Yes, their Ears turn RED with Embarrassment just as soon as they See a Holy Man, or even a Righteous Man: because he Reminds them of their Dietary Sins, and Especially if they are Overweight. Therefore, that is another Good Reason to Fast and Pray: because it Helps such People to Feel Ashamed of themselves, and therefore they might Repent, or Change their Ways of Living. Likewise, whatever Sinner just Looks at a Holy Person, is Immediately Convicted of his Sins: because that Sinner is Reminded of the Laws of God, which are also the Laws of Nature: because they are as ONE, since it was the Creator of all Good Things who Created those Universal Laws.

02-60 [_] You can find a List of more than a hundred Good Reason for Fasting and Praying in my Inspired Book, called: **"HOW to Become a HOLY Man!" (40 Good Reasons WHY People Should FAST and PRAY!) By The Worldwide People's Revolution!® Book 045.** Trust me, if those Good Reasons Inspire you to Fast and Pray, you will come to Understand your Body and Mind Better than ever, just by Imitating your Master, who said: *"The Servant does Well to be Like his Master in all Ways."* Therefore, that is a Good Place to Begin to become Like him, or at least to Understand what he Experienced while Fasting and Praying. Moreover, even if you are an Atheist, and do not Believe in Praying, enough Fasting will Inspire you to do some Praying, which just comes Naturally to the Fasting Person.

— Chapter 03 —

Arguments Against Fasting

03-01 [_] Now, I Hear someone, who is like that Irreverent LOUDMOUTH Sloth-gut Windbag Hole-in-his-Head, say: "O Unelected King, I have read **'HOW to Become a HOLY Man,'** and have come to the Conclusion that you have ADDED LIES to *the Word of God,* and have also TWISTED the *Scriptures,* in order to make them Correspond with your Perverted View of them. Indeed, you have made it out that all People, including myself, must Fast and Pray for 40 Days, like the People of Nineveh did, just because you have Vainly Imagined that such an Act was TRUE Repentance. However, there is nothing within the entire *Bible* that indicates that the People of Nineveh fasted for more than ONE Day, which was the last Day of the 40 Days that Jonah had Warned them about, at which Time a Comet would have Struck the Earth, or perhaps a Meteor would have landed right on the City of Nineveh; but, for sure, no one had to Fast for 40 Days and 40 Nights, consecutively: because most of them would have simply DIED from Hunger: because some People Die from Hunger after missing Meals for just 2 Weeks. However, as if that were not Bad enough, you have made it out that the People of Nineveh fasted without drinking water for 40 days, which would have certainly killed all of them: because a human body cannot go without water, or at least some fruit juices of some kind for any longer than one week: because the kidneys will simply fail, being filled with sticky slime that is somewhat like GLUE! Therefore, such a Radical Fast would be INSANE, even if God Commanded it. Therefore, all of ye false teachers are going to BURN in hellfire forever for thy LIES!" †§

03-02 [_] Well, O Irreverent LOUDMOUTH Sloth-gut Windbag Hole-in-thy-Head, you are in Danger of Hellfire, yourself, just for Suggesting that such a Fast is Impossible: because Moses clearly said that he Fasted for 40 Days and 40 Nights without Eating Foods nor Drinking Waters. (See *Deuteronomy 9:9 and 18,* in any Version that you Like, for the PROOF, even though I much Prefer the New MAGNIFIED Version, which is more Honest.) However, that is not to say that he did not Use any Water at all, in order to take ENEMAS: because he could have done that, even though most *Bibles* do not mention it.

03-03 [_] Nevertheless, it is almost Certain that the People of Nineveh did take Enemas with Water: because they were not used to Fasting, like Moses was. Indeed, Moses had to take a 40-day Fast, just to Enter into the Egyptian School of Higher Learning: because that was their Tradition during that Time, which was Symbolized by the 40 Steps going Up within the Chamber of Light within the Great Pyramid of Cheops {pronounced KEE-ops}. In Fact, Fasting and Praying were Major Parts of the Cultures of almost all Ancient Societies: because they Learned it from Nature and from all of the Holy Prophets and Ascetics. Indeed, the Priests of almost all Tribes Practiced Fasting from India to South Africa, and from Greece to China: because it was Common Knowledge that Fasting would Cure most Diseases, and was certainly the only Daily Remedy for the Previous Day's Overindulgences, which the Ancient Romans also Discovered. Moreover, the Season of LENT has followed a Season of GLUTTONY since Ancient Times, even as the Moslems still continue to hold a Yearly Fast for one whole Month, called Ramadan. In other Words, Fasting has been widely Practiced by almost all Religions; but, especially by Hindus, Buddhists, Jews, Muslims, American Indians, and True Christians. In Fact, the only Religion that I know of, which does not Believe in Fasting, is called the Church of Satan, whose Headquarters is in the Graveyard!

03-04 [_] Now, I Hear someone, who is like a Snake, hiss: "O Peacock, even us Snakes FAST and PRAY for as much as 3 Months between Meals. Likewise, Bears, Squirrels, and many other Animals HIBERNATE, which is FASTING; and even Penguins go for 2 to 3 Months without Eating and without Sleeping in Hibernation: because they Live on their own Fat during that Time. Moreover, Crocodiles Fast for several Months; but, the all-time Record Breakers are the Great WHALES, who normally Fast for 6 Months each Year, while still Nursing their Babies, and while Traveling for thousands of Miles in the Oceans! Therefore, Nature, itself, Teaches us to FAST, or STOP EATING. However, that is not to say that PEOPLE should Fast: because People are HIGHER than Animals, even as it states in *Ecclesiastes 3:19,* which reads: *'For that which befalls the sons of men befalls beasts; as the one dies, so dies the other; yes, they all have one breath, so that a man has no preeminence above a beast: because all is vanity ..."* — *NKJV,* which is a very Sarcastic Statement by King Solomon: because we all Know for a Fact that High Priests are Better than Low Priests, and that Presidents are much Better than VICE Presidents, and that Snakes are *far* Better than Tapeworms! Therefore, Knowing those Facts, it only stands to Reason that People would be Exempt from Fasting: because God gave to People the WISDOM to Invent all Kinds of Drugs, which can be used WISELY, in Order to CURE all Kinds of Ailments, including INSANITY! Yes, I had an Aunt Wretched, who once Claimed to Heal her Broken Leg by taking a certain MediSIN, which she made from Brewing a Dead Snake with 2 Dead Frogs and certain Herbs that she gathered from the Forest, which she said were her 'Secret Herbs.' However, the Doctor Knife said that her Leg just Naturally Healed itself, and also Healed it up CROOKED: beCause she did not put a SPLINT on it; but, only wrapped it with a long Strip of Cloth, which she Soaked in that Snake Brew, which Caused her Leg to get an Infection of the Skin: beCause she did not Change that Bandage for a Month or more! Indeed, it made the entire House STINK like Rotting Flesh; but, Aunt Wretched Insisted that it was doing FINE, in spite of her Great PAINS, for which she took Opium and Heroin, until at last they Buried her in the Little-remembered Unpleasant Valley Slimmetery, where the Worms had a Great Feast on her own Rotting Flesh: because my Uncle Miserable would not Allow her to be Embalmed with Formaldehyde: beCause it would Contaminate her Resurrection, since her Spirit could not Re-enter into such a Defiled Body: because it would be the Equivalent of the Queen of England Living Inside of an Outhouse — you know, one of those Outdoor Toilets or Latrines, which are full of Flies and Capitalist Lies: because no one has Enough Common Sense to put some Sawdust or Peat Moss on Top of their Wastes, in order to Absorb some of the Stink, which can draw Flies for Miles away — all for the Lack of some Limestone Dust and Sawdust. Nevertheless, Aunt Wretched Refused to Fast: because she said that she had House Cleaning to do, and no one else could do it for her: because she had her Particular Method for doing it. Indeed, she would use an Old Sour Dishrag that needed throwing away, which she would Mop all over her Furniture; and afterwards, she would Spray some highly Stinking Perfume all over the House, in order to Camouflage the STINK that she spread around with that Old Sour Dishrag. Moreover, after she would have one of those Stinking Bowel Movements in her Bathroom, she would Spray 3 or 4 Different Kinds of Perfumes all over the Walls, in Order to Try to 'get RID of that Stink,' she said; but, I always thought that it made the whole House Stink just that much more, even though I am a Snake, who normally LIKES Stink. However, her

Stinking Perfumes were Brewed in her own Kitchen, which Smelled somewhat like a Fresh Grave for some Filthy Dog, who got Killed along the Highway during the Heat of Summertime: because Aunt Wretched would bring any Road-killed Varmints Home, and Cook them for our Uncle Miserable, who also Confessed that such Flesh did STINK; but, the Flavor of it at Mealtime made it well Worth it to Tolerate it, even if he had to hold his Nose Closed, until he got it into his Mouth. Furthermore, they had 3 Fat Children, who also liked to Cook, until they got too Fat to do so; and then the whole Family began to go to one of those 'All-you-can-Eat' Buffets, where they Stuffed themselves, Daily, with one ENORMOUS Meal of Hog Slop and Dog Foods, which STRETCHED OUT their Stomachs and Intestines beyond Belief, and made all of them look like Pregnant Cows. Nevertheless, they were a very Happy Family, who always had something Funny to say: because it was Necessary, in Order to Distract their Minds from the Realities of Life. Indeed, if any one of them had ever taken a Good Look at him or herself in the Mirror of Truths, he or she would have surely Fainted at the Sight of it: because they all Carried BIG BAGS of Cellulite on their Hips and Thighs, and had other Bags of Puss under their Eyes; but, it never crossed their Minds that they should FAST: because the Unholy Church of Graceful Sinners never Mentioned it: because People like my Aunt Wretched and Uncle Miserable might be Offended by all such Words as 'FAT and CELLULITE,' even though the *Bible* clearly states that *'The Wrath of God came upon them, and Killed the **Fattest** of them, and Smote Down the Choicest Men of Israel.'* — *Psalm 78:31, RKJV.* Indeed, everyone Knows that Fat People Suffer with more Ailments than any of us Slender Snakes: because their Internal Organs are Overloaded with too much Slime and FAT. However, because of that Fat, all such People can Fast with EASE: beCause they are not Afraid of getting too Skinny, nor Dying from Hunger, like some Skinny Person might be. In Fact, they can easily Fast for 6 Months on nothing but a Quart of Fresh Fruit Juice each Day, and Feel Good: because their Bodies can get Sufficient Nourishment from their Fat." †§‡§§

03-05 [_] Well, O Snake, in spite of your Long Sarcastic Statements, you make more Sense than some People whom I know of, who Imagine that they are much Better than Jesus Christ and Moses, among many other Holy Prophets, who all Fasted OFTEN: because it is the only Way that a Person can get Close to God: beCause the Holy Spirit does not Live within Unclean Temples, as I pointed out in: **"HOW to Become a HOLY Man!" (40 Good Reasons WHY People Should FAST and PRAY!) By The Worldwide People's Revolution!®** Book 045.

03-06 [_] Now, I Hear someone, who is like a Frog, croak: "O Peacock, I Hibernate each Year, during the Winter Months; but, there is a World of DIFFERENCE between *Fasting* and *Hibernating:* beCause, during Hibernation, all Systems of the Body SLOW DOWN, and nearly STOP; but, during Fasting, a Body can actually keep on Working. In Fact, I know of People who have taken long Walks while Fasting, and have even Bragged about how Far that they could go on nothing but AIR Power, while others — such as Paul Bragg — have Bragged about how Far that they could go on nothing but Distilled Water and Air Power. Indeed, Old Man Paul Bragg and a Class of Young College Students went on a Self-inflicted Forced March across the Desert in Death Valley, Nevada, during the Heat of the Summer; and all of the College Students, who were in Prime Athletic Shape, FELL OUT, while Paul Finished the March in Good Spirits, and then turned around and Marched himself back to the Starting Line 3 Days later — not even Stopping to Sleep! Therefore, it could be that Elijah Ate those 2 Meals of Angel Food Cake, which the Angel Baked for him, and Marched for 40 Days unto Mount Horrible, which was apparently a very long ways from the Land of Israel; but, I Doubt that he did not Drink any Water after he got there. In Fact, he probably Drank an entire Barrel of Bud-stupido Beer when he got there." †‡

03-07 [_] Well, O Frog, you completely Misunderstood what is written within your *Bible:* because the Wording is not Exactly Understandable, or Clear: because it was written in such a way as to be Deliberately Misleading, so that Unclean People like you could Imagine that such Foods actually Nourished Elijah for 40 Days, or else he could not have Lived for so Long while Fasting. {See the Correct Translation in: **"HOW to Become a HOLY Man,"** which makes it Clear in *First Kings 19:8,* which Reveals that Elijah Ate those 2 Meals of Fruit Cake, and went to Mount Horeb during a short Time, and continued to Fast for the next 40 Days. After all, Mount Horeb was only 2 Day's Journey from where he was in the Wilderness when he Prayed to Die, while sitting under that Juniper Tree: because we know where the Juniper Trees START and STOP Growing in that Desert. Indeed, you can Consult with Geologists, Phytologists, Botanists, and Paleontologists for that Information, if you Question what I tell you.

03-08 [_] Now, I Hear someone, who is like a Cockroach, say: "O Peacock, you might as well Consult with a Garbologist for that Information: because Climates have Radically Changed since the Days of Elijah. For Example, the Great Saharan Desert was once Forested with Juniper and Pine Trees, as Scientists have Proven. Indeed, our own American Petrified Forest in Arizona, was once a LIVING FOREST, or else those Petrified Redwood Trees could not have gotten there, even if Noah's Flood washed them over there from Californicate." †‡

03-09 [_] Well, O Cockroach, there is no use in Speculating about what Happened, or did not Happen, thousands of Years Ago: because, "too much Water has Washed Under the Bridge since then," as they say. Indeed, if just one small Piece of Information were Missing from your Nolij, you could completely Misjudge such Subjects, and even come up with Irrational Conclusions like Modern Scientists have come up with, who do their Best to Eliminate the Awesome Power of the Divine Creator from all of their Equations — not to mention what Holy Angels could have done for the FUN of it. After all, if you were an Angel, and you had 6 billion People to Play with their Minds, would you not be Tempted to do Strange Things for them, in order to get them to THINK? For Example, the Petrified Redwood Forest that was found in Arizona, could have come from Redwood Trees that once Grew in Arizona at a Time when the entire North and South American Continents were Connected with Europe and Africa, some 5,000 Years Ago. However, what does any of that have to do with **"The Proper RULES for FASTING"**?

03-10 [_] And he Answers, "I just Thought that it was something that you might be Interested in, whether or not it is Connected with Fasting."

— Chapter 04 —

WHO should NOT Fast?

04-01 [ ] Well, as I wrote in: **"HOW to Become a HOLY Man,"** there are certain People who should NOT be Fasting — such as Pregnant Mothers, little Babies, and People who are so Skinny and Weak that they are already Starving for Nourishment. Indeed, such Mothers might LOSE their Babies: because Fasting can Cause Natural Abortions in Pregnant Mothers. However, even if such Abortions do not take place, Fasting can Cause Mothers to Lose their Teeths, or at least Weaken their Teeths: because that Nourishment is Transferred from the Mothers to their little Babies, in order to give to them a Chance to Live, even if the Mothers Die. (See *Genesis 35.*)

04-02 [ ] Nevertheless, both the Mother and the Child can become Malnourished, and end up with Physical and/or Mental Defects. Therefore, if you are Fasting for the Purpose of Aborting a Baby by God's Natural and Authorized Means, make Sure that you go on through with it unto the END: beCause a Deformed Baby could Mean an Eternal Heartache or Great Regret — that is, IF you have gone on a Long Fast of 3 Weeks or more: because a Short Fast on one Week or less might not Cause any Harm, neither to you, nor to your Child. However, it is not Recommended that any Pregnant Mother should Fast, unless she has no other Rational Choice: because of getting Severely Injured, or because of getting some Sickness or Disease, whereby she loses her Appetite.

04-03 [ ] Therefore, it is also Recommended that all Pregnant Mothers should be ISOLATED or Quarantined from Society, in order to AVOID "Catching" Colds, Flqz, and Contagious Diseases of Various Kinds — such as Measles, Mumps, Chicken Pox, Diphtheria, and so on. In other Words, STAY AT HOME WHERE YOU BELONG, as your *Bible* Teaches; and do your Socializing AFTER your Baby is a Year or 2 Old, if you must go Looking for Diseases among Sick People, who seem to be Magnetized to certain Churches or Congregations of Sick Idiots. (See *Titus 2.*)

04-04 [ ] Indeed, you could hardly find Sicker People than you would find at most American Churches: because they have Systematic PARTIES and FEASTS for FOOLS; and you can Hear them Sniffing and Coughing during almost every Meeting during the Wintertime: because they come to Church Meetings for Prayers, in Order to be Healed from such Sicknesses, and to Hear Flattering LIES — such as that Lie about *"... nothing entering into the mouth can defile a man,"* which is taken OUT of Context with all of the Teachings of Jesus Christ, who was no Ignorant Fool, who Knew for a Fact that if anyone should Eat Enough Poison, he or she would DIE; but, at the least, he or she would certainly get SICK: because only HOLY People do not get Sick, even if they Eat Poisonous Foods: because their Bodies can Handle it, and Eliminate it. (See *Mark 16:18,* and Understand that Jesus was speaking about True Believers, ONLY; and not the General Public, who do NONE of those Things that are Listed in *Mark 16.*)

04-05 [_] For Example, my Brother Vern Unknowingly Ate some Poisoned Canned Fishes many Years Ago, and within 5 Minutes he VOMITED THEM OUT, and therefore he did not get Sick, nor even Feel Bad afterwards; but, that same Can of Fishes might have Killed other People, whose Bowels would not be Working so Good, in Order to Save them: because they have been putting Various Kinds of Poisons into their Stomachs for many Years, and have Abused their Stomachs with Various Kinds of Concoctions in their Suicidal Kitchens, whereby almost every Meal is a Big Gamble with their Lives!

04-06 [_] Nevertheless, do not Allow me to Discourage you from Eating Dog Foods nor Hog Slop, if that is what you Desire to Eat: because, if that is your Desire, you probably NEED such Foods, just to Humble you for your Foolishness. Yes, you are somewhat like the Prodigal Son, who must Experiment with your Lusts, in Order to Discover how BAD they are; but, afterwards, you will be quite Willing to take a long FAST, just to Recover from your Self-indulgences. In other Words, you might Eat like a Hog, TODAY; but, in the Morning you will be Ready to REPENT.

04-07 [_] Indeed, I have known People who did it, DAILY, and are still doing it: because they do not have any Clue as to HOW to STOP IT! And other People Eat, and then Vomit, Daily: because they do not Know HOW to STOP IT, until they get "Counseling" from "Professionals," who themselves are also Addicted to this Food, or to that Drink, or to Smoke, or to some other Bad Habits: because the Devil has a Multitude of Ways and Means, in Order to bring us down to his Hellish Condition. Indeed, one of his Favorite Methods is by Means of PORNOGRAPHY, which he uses on People who are Addicted to Beautiful Bodies, who cannot Resist having Longing Desires to have Sex with such Bodies: because they have been Greatly DEPRIVED of such Sensual Pleasures, or because they have just had Enough of it to Crave more of it.

04-08 [_] Indeed, there is nothing on this Earth that is as Beautiful and Enticing as a Young Healthy Naked Body, which was *"... made in the Image of God."* However, none of those "Evil Things" nor Lustful Desires have any Effect on Babies, who are as Innocent as little Lambs, who are not Deprived of Love, Attention, nor Affection; and they Certainly have no Desire to Smoke nor use Drugs. No, they do not even know what Lust Means, let alone have any Longing Desire to Jump into Bed with some Painted Stinking Skunk; and, like all Babies, they only need to be Loved, Fed, Cleaned, and kept Warm or Cool and Comfortable: because their Desires are very Limited.

04-09 [_] Nevertheless, you can See that many Fat little Babies are already on the Road to Hell, as they say: because they are Unnaturally FAT: beCause of being Deprived of Natural Wholesome Foods, and especially Sweet Juicy Fruits. Indeed, many American Babies are Fed Junk Foods by Fat Parents, who are Addicted to all such Foods and Sugar Water. Moreover, it has been Reported that more than 50 percent of Americans are now Overweight, and 50% of those are OBESE, which Means that they weigh anywhere from 100 to 500 Pounds too much.

04-10 [_] Now, I Hear a very Fat Person, say: "O Slender Peacock, many of us Fat People are Suffering with Diabetes; and therefore, we cannot Fast: because, if we just Miss a single Meal, we might go into Seizures, and even DIE from it! Therefore, HOW are we supposed to Fast?"

04-11 [_] Well, my Friend, it Appears that you have gotten yourself into a Real Living Hell, from which only God can Deliver you. However, you could just CHANGE your DIET, and begin to Eat all-Natural WHOLE Foods — such as Brown Rice, rather than White Polished Rice; and you could Eat Homemade Whole Wheat Bread with Real Honey, as Opposed to White Refined Flour with Refined Sugar and Various Kinds of Poisonous Chemicals in Commercial Breads; but, beCause of so much Waste Matter within your Bowels, those Foods would not be Satisfying, and they might even Cause you to have another Seizure: because a Muscular *Seizure* is the Body's Method of TRYING to Eliminate something that it cannot otherwise Eliminate, which it Desperately Wants to get RID OF by Violent Contractions of the Muscles.

04-12 [_] Therefore, with your Doctor's Permission, you might Experiment for 6 Months with a Diet of nothing but Fresh Green Leaves and Homemade Whole Wheat Bread, which you have Soaked in some Kind of Fruit Juice, just to Discover whether or not you get Tired of such a Diet, and therefore Eat less and less of it. Indeed, the Maya Indians had a SOLO WHOLE CORN DIET for any Person who committed any Crime, or who otherwise needed Correcting: because they Ate less and less of that Whole Corn, or Maize, until at last they were FASTING: because they could not Tolerate it any longer; and then, behold, it was not long before they completely Recovered from whatever "Possessed" them. Yes, "the Demon Spirits left them within a Year, or so," they Reported: because they were simply FASTING, or Abstaining to some Degree from Eating certain Foods, which Allowed their Bodies to Eliminate whatever Unwanted Waste Matter was Accumulated within them.

04-13 [_] Likewise, you must do something to LOSE your Enormous Appetite, even if you must go on that Whole Corn Diet — that is, on Natural Mature Organically-grown WHOLE Corn, which you can Boil in Salted Water, Daily, for about one Month, and then leave the Salt OUT of the Water after that, in Order to Discover how TASTELESS that Corn IS *without* Salt nor Spices. Yes, you will LOATHE it, or HATE to Think of it: because of its Foul Taste, unless you only Eat such a Small Amount of it that you are Hungry for it, which will be about one Cup of it.

04-14 [_] However, such a Poor Diet is NOT very Healthy for any Body: because you will be Starving for Real Foods, which are Fresh Raw Fruits and Clean Green Leaves and a few Raw Nuts, which you can also LIMIT to just ONE Cup of Dried Fruit, 2 Cups of Cooked Greens, and about 4 to 10 Nuts — such as Walnuts, Pecans, or Almonds; and only Eat ONE Meal during the Morning, at 10 O'clock; and another Meal at 6 P.M. Meanwhile, you can Exercise by going for long Walks, except that such Walks will not Satisfy your Natural Demand for Real Accomplishments — such as Building your own House, Furniture, or something that you and others can SEE and Appreciate: because such Accomplishments are just as Necessary as Foods and Drinks, when it comes to Satisfying the Soul, which is made up of a Body AND a Spirit.

04-15 [_] In Fact, the American Deathstyle, itself, can be Rightly Blamed for the Poor Lifestyle of most Obese Americans, who have Jobs like Policemen and Firemen, who sit around for most of the Day, waiting for Evil Things to Happen, which Naturally gives to them Evil Appetites: because of their IDLE Minds, Hands and Bodies. Therefore, no matter what you do for a Living, you must Try to keep your Mind Occupied with something other than FOODS and Drinks, which Means that you will also have to SHUT OFF that Television with all of its *Enchantments,* or *Repetitious Chants,* which Advertise Hamburgers, Pizzas, Iced-creams, Candies, Cookies, Cakes,

Drugs, Cars, Pickup Trucks, and whatever is for Sale: because it continually Reminds you to EAT! (See *Isaiah 47:9,* and Remember that *Sorceries* are *Druggeries,* and *Enchantments* are *Advertisements* for those Addictive Things.)

04-16 [_] Indeed, you must think of yourself as being in a very Dangerous and Horrible Condition, for which you must become DESPERATE, and even REFUSE to *Think* about Foods: because it could easily KILL you! Yes, you must set your Mind on Spiritual Things, or at least on some Work that you can Do, in Order to Distract your Mind from the Thoughts of Eating and Drinking. However, before you Eat, you should Drink some Fruit Juice, and wait for at least an Hour: because you might Lose your Appetite, and therefore be able to Fast for at least 6 more Hours, before you Drink some more Fresh Fruit Juice or Carrot Juice, or just Eat an Apple, after you Thank the Creator for it: because the Act of Prayer, alone, will Help to REDUCE your Appetite, if you do it with Sincerity.

04-17 [_] Now, I Hear someone, who is like a Walrus, snort: "O Peacock, have you ever Tried to Eat such a Meal with a Handful of Raisins and Nuts, and be Contented with it?"

04-18 [_] Well, O Walrus, I just finished with such a Meal, having some Fresh Homegrown Cucumbers with those Raisins and Nuts, and I found it very Satisfying, except that I need to take a Shower, in Order to Feel Truly Refreshed. Indeed, Unclean Pores in the Skin can make a Person Feel Unsatisfied for a Lack of Oxygen: because the Skin Breathes, being the largest single Organ of the Body, which also Expels Various Kinds of Waste Matter — such as Excess Salt, Beef Broth, Chicken Broth, Grease, Fat, Oil, Cheese, and whatever it might Sweat Out, or Squeeze Out in the Form of Blackheads, Pimples, Boils, and so on. In Fact, the Skin can get a Sore on it, and OOZE Out Puss and Slime for YEARS, as many People have Proven: beCause the Skin provides a Secondary Means of Elimination of Filth, after the Bowels cannot Handle so much Excess Food. Therefore, even Babies SWEAT: because their Bowels are not Able to Eliminate all of the Waste Matter that they should be Able to Eliminate, if they were Saturated with Fresh Raw Fruit Juices, after Feasting on Ripe Mangos and Cherimoyas.

04-19 [_] Now, I Hear someone, who is like an Old Lady, say: "O Peacock, I have a Granddaughter who weighs in at about 450 Pounds (or about 204 Kilograms), even though her Mother and I never got over 140 Pounds (or about 63.5 Kilograms); and she Sweats Profusely, even during a Cool Day; and she is often Sick, after Eating a Meal of Spaghetti and Meat Balls with Tomato Sauce, which Smells just like Vomit, to me: because she sprinkles Cheese or Dried Cow's Puss on Top of it. However, if I should stop Eating, I would just Blow Away: because I only weigh about 90 Pounds, and I am so Weak that I can barely get myself Out of Bed, even though I never Sweat or Perspire. Therefore, what are we supposed to Do, since I cannot Trade my Skinny Bones for my Granddaughter's *Biblical* Tub of Lard? — that is, her Lard is in *Biblical* Proportions, if you know what I Mean!" †

04-20 [_] Well, O Grandma, you have probably noticed that your Granddaughter Eats about 10 Times more than you do, which is WHY that she is so FAT; but, as for Trading any of that Fat for your Skinniness would only make you Weaker: because it is not Healthy Fat, as some Doctor might be able to Demonstrate to you, if you Visit some Hospital where they are Operating on such People: because her Fat is no doubt laced with Harmful Chemicals and Poisons, which

Naturally Accumulate within FATS of all Kinds. For Example, if there are Harmful Chemicals within Nuts and Grains, those Chemicals will be Stored within the Fat or Oil, itself. Therefore, when you Eat something that is Fried or otherwise Cooked with Cottonseed Oil, for Example, you should Understand that you are getting an Unfair Dose of Harmful Chemicals: because Cotton is Sprayed with Deadly Poisons, since no one Supposedly Eats it; but, they do Eat Cottonseed OIL, which has a Legal Amount of Harmful Poisons in it, which is also True for all other "Edible" Oils: because it would be Difficult, if not Impossible, for most Farmers to Grow Foods *without* using certain Pesticides, Herbicides, and Chemical Fertilizers, and still Earn a PROFIT: beCause the Bugs and Pests would Destroy their Crops: because they have Poisoned their Land so much that it does not have any Natural Resistance to such Bugs nor Pests.

04-21 [_] However, we Grew upwards of 40 Bushels of Irish Potatoes last Year, and we did not Discover so much as ONE Potato Bug within the entire Garden, and we did not use any Sprays of any Kind anywhere in the whole Garden! In Fact, the only Enemy that we seem to have, and cannot Control are those Acid Rains, which can easily Ruin an entire Crop.

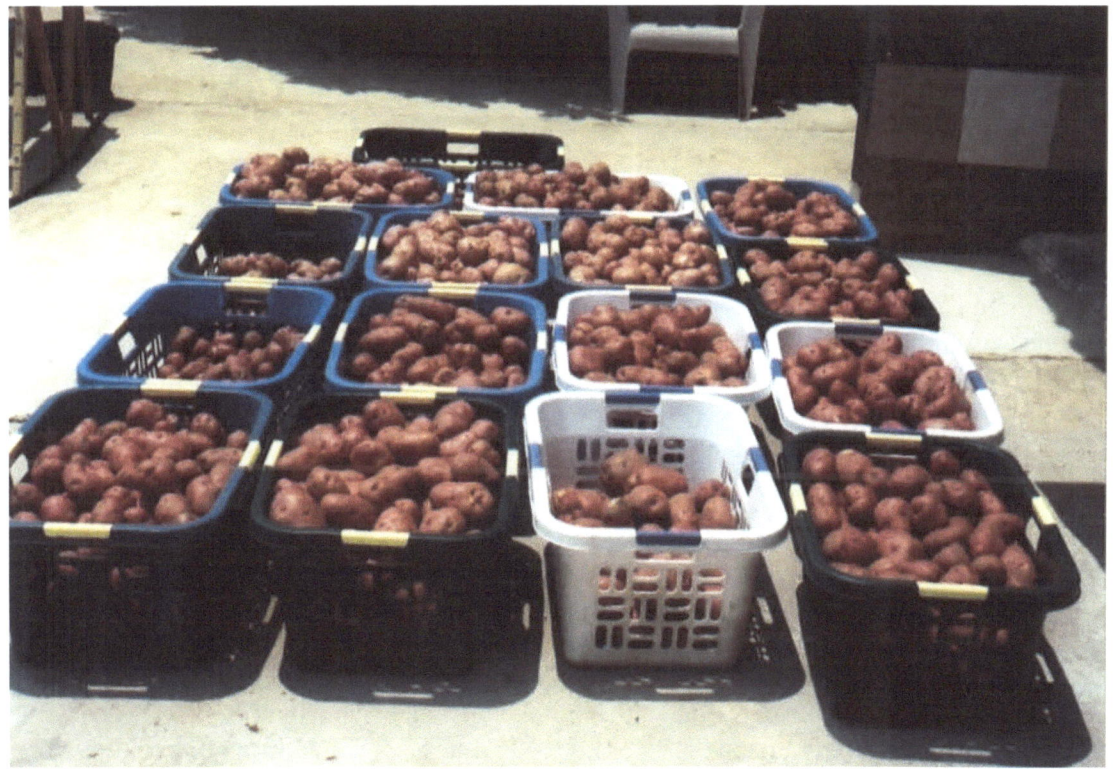

{FOOTNOTE: Here are some of those Irish Potatoes, most of which I put into Canning Jars, along with a couple hundred Butternut Squashes, Onions, and Beans for 2,000 Quarts of Survival Foods. I Harvested all of these Potatoes alone with a Digging Fork during just one Morning, and Washed them in Cold Spring Water, and Sorted all of them in the Shade of my large Fig Tree during the same Afternoon, and put them in Storage, and then Moved them Out of our 98% Rock House Storage Room for this Photo, and then Moved them back into the House by Muscle Power. None of them were Lost. I also gave 10% of them to the Salvation Army in Texarkana for a Tithe Offering: so that we would be Blest with a hundredfold more the next Year.}

— Chapter 05 —

Who SHOULD Fast?

05-01 [_] Well, according to the *Bible,* the People and the Animals of the entire City of Nineveh, consisting of more than 120,000 People, plus perhaps a million Animals, Fasted for 40 Days and 40 Consecutive Nights, while they Patiently Waited to Discover whether or not God would Spare them or Destroy them. {See *The New MAGNIFIED Version (NMV)* of that Story in: **"The Gospel According to our Elected King!" (The Good News from the Most Modern Perspective!) By The Worldwide People's Revolution!®** Book 013. Chapter 06 contains one of the Best Sermons in the Whole World, if not *the* Best.}

05-02 [_] In other Words, no one was Excused from that Great Fast, which was Conducted by Jonah, who gave a Special Sermon to them, in order to Explain HOW to do it Correctly. (See also *Matthew 12:41, King James Version.*) In other Words, Jonah had a lot more to say than was Recorded within most *Holy Bibles:* beCause it would have been Bad for Business, even as all other Truths are Bad for Capitalist Businesses, which Rely on Addictions.

05-03 [_] Nevertheless, there is no mention made of any Person nor Animal that was Excused from that Fast, which was perhaps the All-time Record in World History of Repentance: because the entire City Repented, minus none: because the Option was DEATH! Yes, the King would have had their Heads Removed, if they had Decided NOT to Repent: because he Commanded them to do so; and they Obeyed, and were thus Saved from Destruction, being Physiologically *"Born Again,"* in spite of Diabetes or whatever else might have Ailed them at that Time. In other Words, one Wise Honest King Saved their Lives, for which they must have Thanked him, and also Wrote their own Autobiographies about their Experiences with Fasting. †‡

05-04 [_] Now, I Hear someone, who is like a Skeptic, say: "O Peacock, how does anyone Know for Sure that the People of Nineveh would have been Destroyed, if they had NOT Repented? Indeed, what was it that Persuaded them that such Destruction could come?"

05-05 [_] Well, O Skeptic, that is a very Good Question, since most People would simply Scoff at the Idea of Fasting for 40 Days and 40 Nights; but, no one in his nor her Right Mind can Honestly Deny that most Americans Desperately Need to FAST, just like Nineveh, lest the Men of Nineveh should rise up in Judgment with this Generation of Evildoers, and Condemn it: because we have NOT Repented. Therefore, when Americans Witness the Power of God, which will be Revealed by Means of Various Kinds of Miracles during these Last Days, they will also come to Realize that if they do not Repent, they will also be Destroyed, even as Babylon, Zidon, Tyre, Sodom, Gomorra, and many other Ancient Cities and Kingdoms were Destroyed by one Means or another: beCause they would not REPENT.

05-06 [_] Now, I Hear someone, who is like that Irreverent LOUDMOUTH Sloth-gut Windbag Hole-in-Thy-Head, say: "O Peacock, the Thief who Died on the Cross beside of Christ did NOT have Time to Repent, like Nineveh: because he Died that same Day. Moreover, Jesus said that he would be with him in Paradise that same Day. Therefore, you are Teaching a FALSE Doctrine, for which you will no doubt go straight to Hell: because God HATES all such LIES! In Fact, it is Doubtful that the People of Nineveh fasted for more than 2 or 3 Days, just before the 40 Days of Jonah's Prophecy should be completed: because it Required 30 Days or more for the uninspired words of Jonah to reach the King: because Nineveh was a very LARGE City of more than 75 Miles across it, which Required a whole Day's Journey, just to cross it by Stagecoach, and perhaps 4 Day's Journey by Oxpower with a Cart. In fact, if you had been Living in Nineveh, and some Ignorant Fool came along, and all that he said was: *'Yet 40 Days, and Nineveh shall be Overthrown,'* you would say that such a Person must be CRAZY: because he did not give to you any REASON for such an Overthrow. Therefore, he might as well have Danced on the Head of a Pin, or Swallowed an Elephant's Head, as far as most of us are concerned: because no one can Fast for 40 Days and 40 Nights, even if he or she takes Enemas, Daily: because he or she will DIE from THIRST, even as I have Proven for myself: because I have fasted for just one Week, and it seemed as though I would Die from Thirst, even though I did not take any Enemas: because I was Ignorant concerning such Subjects. Nevertheless, I am not going to Try to undertake another Dry Fast: because I might Die. However, the whole Doctrine is FALSE: because the Thief who Died on the Cross beside of Jesus Christ did NOT do any Fasting; but, he simply said, *'Lord, remember me when you come into your kingdom.'* Therefore, Jesus said to him, *'Truly I say to you Today, that you shall be with me in Paradise; but, first, you must be Born Again, in Order for God to Test your Spirit, in Order to Discover if you are Sincere. But, as for this other Criminal, he will be with me Today, when I Visit those Spirits that were Living before the Great Flood, who have been Reserved in Chains of Darkness, until now, at which Time most of them will Repent and be Saved: because they will only have to say, "O Lord, we Believe in thee; yes, we Accept thee as our Anointed Savior, even though we are not Willing to Do anything that thou might Teach to us: because we do not Accept thee as our Master nor Savior." Indeed, they will not have to Beg for Forgiveness for their Sins, nor even Confess that they had any Dietary Sins at all: because there is no such a Thing as Dietary Sins, since nothing can Defile a Person that enters into his nor Mouth, even if he or she consumes 10 times more than he or she needs for Nourishment: because God Judges by the Heart, not by the Appearance of the Stomach that drags along the Ground in the Mud like a Hog's Stomach. After all, look at Moses for a Good Example, who came down from Mount Sinai as Fat as a Hog just after Fasting for 40 Days on Biscuits and Gravy, as it states in Poodersnook 13:45, which is just after Deuteronomy 9:9, and 18. Yes, you can read it for yourself, Peter, in Order to Discover that it does not matter if you weigh as much as a Walrus or Whale, just as long as you Confess that you Believe in my Name, which is Yak Jez Yaknackeryak, Son of BeLIEal, the Third. Indeed, the First Yaknackeryak was Moses, himself, who wrote 5 books full of LIES, which only a Fool would Believe: because it is Impossible for any Person to Fast for more than a Day or 2, and even then such a Person might Cheat just a little, by licking on an Ice-cream Cone, sneaking some Candy, or Drinking a Beer; but, for sure, nothing in that Bible can be Trusted: because it was written by People who never Actually Fasted for one whole Day during their Lives, or else they would have Discovered that it is Impossible! Nevertheless, beside all of that, we are Saved by GRACE, not by Works, like Fasting: because it Requires a LOT of Work, in Order to lie in Bed and FAST: because you have to fix Meals for your whole Family, and even Wash the Clothes by Hand: because, just as soon as you begin to Fast, the entire Family suddenly comes up with a thousand Projects that need to be Done! Therefore, it Requires far more Work than most People can Imagine — not to mention those Prayers, which you must say while CRAWLING up to the Top of*

Mount Pizgah on your Stomach, like a Snake! Yes, you must Repeat the Lord's Prayer ten thousand times per Day, which Requires far more WORK than most People can Imagine! Nevertheless, most People also Cheat on that, and just Mumble something like this, "O Lord, please look upon me in my State of Poverty, and Understand that I need millions of dollars, so that I might buy a 40-room Mansion with all of the latest Gadgets, so that I might be Happy: because Happiness comes from Possessing all Kinds of Vain Things, of which the World has an Endless Supply: because thousands of People are Inventing new Things each Year, many of which become Popular; and therefore, we must have them. Yes, O Lord, I BEG YOU TO PLEASE make me Rich, so that I can Obtain Peace of Mind: because of having Enough Money, in Order to REST from all of my Toils and Labors: because of Hiring Servants at Minimum Wages, in Order to do the Work for me: because that is what I would Desire that some Rich Person should do for me, if I were one of those Low Class Poor People from some Foreign Country, who cannot even speak this Language, who does not Deserve more than a Mud Hut to Live in." †§‡§§ And thus it shall be during the Last Days, whenever People Attempt to Fast.'

05-07 [_] "Now, therefore, O Proud Peacock, there is no Good Reason for any Person to Repent by Means of Fasting nor Praying: because God does not Require it of thee, since none of the Holy Prophets did it; nor do any of our Modern Medical Doctors do it: because Fasting and Praying could not Save them from their Dietary Sins, neither: because they would have their Heads under the Sheets of the Hospital Beds, licking on some Chocolate Pudding, in Secret! Yes, former President Bill Adulterous Lying Clinton could Teach to us a few Things about Dietary Sins, except that the Rev. Dr. Billy Graham says that he Forgives Bill, even though Bill did not Ask for Forgiveness: because it is no Sin to have Oral Sex, which is Clean Sex, just as long as you do it in Secret in the Oval Orifice, in the Little White OUTHOUSE, in Washington, District of Corruption. Therefore, the Question is NOT, 'Should we Fast and Pray until we Overcome our Sins?' but, rather, 'Should God Apologize for Commanding us to Do something that is Impossible?' Indeed, the whole Idea is INSANE: because that Thief on the Cross did not have 40 Days, in Order to do his Fasting, like Nineveh had; and he certainly did not get Born Again: because *'it was appointed unto men once to die, and after that the judgment,'* as it states in *Hebrews 9:27,* which Means that the Thief on the Cross must have also Risen Up from the Dead that same Day, in Order for him to get into the Paradise with Eyeballs, Ears, Nostrils, and a Body that might Sense that it is Alive — or else there was no Reason for the Resurrection of Jesus Christ, who did not have to get back into his Body, since a Body is not Required, in Order to Live forever; or else, Jesus would have said, *'I will see you while in the Spirit in Paradise, Today, just after I Visit those Spirits that are still in Prison, who have been Suffering with Aches and Pains in their Muscles and Bones ever since Noah, when they Died in the Great Flood, and the Sharks Ate their Bodies; but, not Enough of them, in Order to get Rid of them: because it would bring the Word of God into Confusion, who Promised that he would Send those Spirits to Prison, where they could be Spiritually Chained up for the next 3,000 Years, in Darkness, where they could neither See, Hear, Smell, Taste, nor Touch anyone: because Spirits do not need Bodies, in Order to Suffer with Headaches, Leg-aches, Backaches, Sore Throats, Colds, Flues, and Diarrheas of the Mouth. No, Spirits do not even need Hearts nor Brains, which is WHY that Jesus had to somehow get back into his Body after he was Crucified, in Order to DECEIVE US: because, if Spirits do not need Bodies, in order to Suffer, as those Spirits did for 3,000 Years since Noah, then Jesus would not have needed a Body, neither: because he is Greater than those Spirits, if ye know what I Meaneth. In other Words, the whole Doctrine of Immortal Spirits is just*

INSANE: because a Spirit without a Body is DEAD; and therefore, ye are all Dead.' See *Cladclickerdome 34:45.* Nevertheless, I am not asking you to Believe any of those silly things, O Peacock: because you could probably Prove most of them to be WRong, or Insane; but, I am only asking you to consider how CRAZY it is to think that we Americans could Repent by Means of Fasting and Praying for 40 Long Days and 40 Dreadful Nights, like the People of Nineveh did, considering how GLUTTONOUSLY FAT that we American HOGS are, including thyself, who must Weigh at least 150 Pounds, when John the Baptist only Weighted 90 Pounds." †§‡§§

05-08 [_] Well, O Irreverent LOUDMOUTH Sloth-gut Windbag Hole-in-Thy-Head, I am not going to Waste my Time nor anyone else's Time with any Explanations for your Extremely Sarcastic Statements, which you have Woven Together like a Spider's Web. However, I would like to point out that Fasting is the Opposite of Working: because it is Abstaining from all Works; and no such Repetitious Prayers will have any Effect with God, who Thinks of all such People as Heathen Idiots, who Vainly Imagine that God is as Stupid as they are.

05-09 [_] Remember this: **"When you Learn the Truth about Fasting, and then Practice it According to the Rules, you will come to Know for a Fact that it is a Provable Truth: beCause it will set you Free from Aches, Pains, Sores, Itches, Burns, Wounds, Doctor Bills, Pills, Lotions, Potions, Snake-oil Remedies, and whatever is found for Sale by Selfish Drug Pushers and Greedy Capitalist Hogs." — The other Apostle Paul**

05-10 [_] I have Heard that if a Diabetic Person simply Changes his or her Diet, and consumes only Wholesome Natural Foods, with nothing Refined, that his or her Diabetes will simply Disappear within 2 to 3 Weeks, if he or she is Young; and, within 2 to 3 Months, if he or she is Old. Therefore, it apparently Works Well for certain People, which is Worth a Test on your own Body, if you are Bold enough to Eat with Jesus Christ and his Disciples, none of whom had Access to any Highly-refined Garbage Foods in Gross Grocery Stores. In other Words, try Eating nothing but RAW Sweet Immature Whole Corn from an All-Mineral Organic Garden for a Month or 2, and Discover just how GOOD it is, just as it is. I Mean that you should Stand in the Corn Patch, and Shuck the Cob and Eat it Immediately, whenever you get Hungry, even as any Wild Animal would just Naturally do. Moreover, if it is Good Corn, it will be Satisfying, all by itself, without Adding any Salt, Pepper, Butter, nor anything else. Furthermore, you will Dread the Day when the Sweet Corn runs out, and there is no more to Harvest. Therefore, be sure to plant New Seeds every Week, beginning in early Springtime, and Remove the Corn Stalk after you have Harvested the Corn Cobs from it, which you can put in your Compost Pile, or use it to Mulch around the other Corn Plants. However, if you are Afraid of a Mono Diet of nothing but Sweet Corn, then Plant some Onion Sets to munch on with the Corn. English Peas will be ready to Eat long before the Corn, if you Plant the Pea Seeds a Month before the last Frost, since they Tolerate Frosts, and seem to do Better with Frosts. Moreover, even if they completely Freeze Off, they will Spring Back and Beg for more Frosts: beCause they are Determined to LIVE!

— Chapter 06 —

How to PREPARE for a Fast

06-01 [_] Some Professing "Experts" Suggest that there is no Need to PREPARE for a Fast: because that would somehow be "Cheating God of his Glory," as if God Delighted himself with our Sufferings and Self-inflicted Torments. Indeed, they say that the more Difficult that it is for us to Fast, the more Sorry that we will Feel for having Abused ourselves by committing Dietary Sins; and therefore, because of Suffering while Fasting, we will be less Apt to commit those same Dietary Sins again: because our Suffering will Help us to Remember our Dietary Sins, and thus Help to Prevent them.

06-02 [_] However, I say that most People will Suffer Enough, even if they do their Fasting Properly: because they have Eaten so many Unnatural Foods, which have Caused Gall Stones, Kidney Stones, Arthritis, Gout, Cancers, and whatever, which will probably put them in Pains to some Degree, which will be Sufficient Torment. Moreover, if such People DREAD to do any Fasting, and then they Discover that it is Extremely Painful, they are not likely to do any more of it; but, if they Discover that it is relatively EASY, they are more Apt to do it more often: because they are Encouraged to Fast.

06-03 [_] Therefore, let each Person Decide which Way is the Best Way for him or herself, and then stick with it, until he or she is Convinced. After all, if you cannot Learn the Truth from me, you can Learn it from Personal Experiences, or from the Experiences of other Ascetics, such as Moses, Elijah, Daniel, Peter, Paul, and John.

06-04 [_] However, for those Wise People, who Want to Learn it from me, the Best Way for a Person to Prepare for a Fast, is to Change his or her Diet for at least one Week, at which Time he or she should Eat nothing but Laxative Foods, even if they Cause a Diarrhea, or the "RUNS," which will Empty the Bowels to some Degree, which will make Sure that such a Person does not Die from some Blockage within his or her Bowels.

06-05 [_] In other Words, the PIPES that are called Bowels, will be SWEPT OUT to some Degree by the Roughage that is Eaten. Therefore, in Order to Assist the Bowels to get Thoroughly Swept Out, you should Eat mostly Coleslaw without the Mayonnaise, which can be Substituted with Ripe (but not Overripe) Avocadoes, Shredded Carrots, Chopped Celery, Diced Green Onions, Bell Peppers, Raisins, Diced Cucumbers, and some Natural Soy Sauce for Seasoning, if you like it. You can mix some Lime Juice with the mashed Avocadoes to keep them from turning Dark. You can also use some Dulse, instead of Soy Sauce, which is Naturally Salty; but, only if you are feeling Rich: because the Dulse is very Expensive, being a Dignified Sea Weed, which might also contain Sea Shells and Parts of Sea Creatures, including Dung. However, properly Washed and Cleaned Dulse is difficult to Surpass for Flavor and Satisfaction. Indeed, the Dulse is very Rich with Minerals, and will Satisfy your Hunger for Sodium, while at the same Time it will Greatly Flavor your Coleslaw.

06-06 [_] Moreover, if you get Tired of that "Boring Diet," you can Trade it for another Diet that is similar with Different Flavors. For Example, you can Eat Steamed Broccoli, which is Dipped in Avocado Dressing with a little Lime Juice and Soy Sauce with Chopped Green Onions and Red Bell Peppers, which will be about half as Laxative as the Coleslaw; but, it will Work Well in your Bowels, if you have another Meal of Fresh Raw Fruits, or Dried Fruits during the Morning; or, at least Drink a half-gallon of Fruit Juice — such as Orange or Apple Juice — during the Day, which will Help to Loosen Up your Stool or Feces, which is called *"Dung"* in the *Holy Bible,* which might Sound Nasty to some Sophisticated People, who do not like the Smell of their own Dung: beCause it STINKS, while that of Holy People does NOT Stink, and is perfectly Good Fertilizer for Fruit Trees and Nut Trees, which should be Covered with some Topsoil, Immediately, in order to get Maximum Benefits from it as a Fertilizer, which will make the Fruits much more Fragrant, Sweet, and Satisfying, which is God's Gardening Plan, which Ignorant Fools have not Improved on by the Inventions of Chemical Fertilizers, which are Missing many Important Elements that are Necessary for Healthy Happy Gardening. Trust me, God's Plan is the Best; but, it also Requires RULES. {See www.Amazon.com for: **"The LUSCIOUS All-Mineral Organic Method of Gardening!" (HOW to Grow DELICIOUS Satisfying Foods for Potential Kingz and Kweenz in Swanky PALACES!)**, Book 021, plus: **"Did God or Satan Ordain Medical Doctors??" (Ask Huck Finn and/or Nigger Jim: because neither Tom Sawyer nor Judge Thatcher would Know!) By The Worldwide People's Revolution!®** Book 022.}

06-07 [_] Nevertheless, if that Diet seems to be too Radical: because of getting the "RUNS," it only means that it is Time for you to Fast: beCause your Body is Ready for an Elimination of Toxic Filth. In other Words, if you Eat that Coleslaw for 2 or 3 Days, and get a Diarrhea, the Time to begin your Fast is following that Diarrhea, which you can Encourage by Drinking some Fruit Juices, in Order to make SURE that your Bowels are EMPTIED, as much as it is Possible during that Time: because it will make your Fasting rather easy: because there will be *less* Ancient Morbid Matter within your Bowels to Torment you.

06-08 [_] However, you must Remember that the Pockets of your Bowels will still Retain a certain Amount of Filth, which will continue to Torment you, until it is *Thoroughly* Removed by Fasting and Flushing Out your Bowels. Therefore, it Requires much Patience, Time, and Persistence, in Order to Accomplish your Goal, which is Holiness of Mind, Spirit, and Body, which cannot be Obtained without MUCH Fasting and Praying: because it Required many Years of Self-abuse, in Order to Accumulate that Morbid Filth that is now Lodged within you, which is Tormenting you, which Normally Accumulates very Slowly, even as it is Eliminated very Slowly; but, Surely, if you are Persistent and Determined to get it ALL Out of you, whereby you will at last be set Free with a Capital F, at which Time you will be Free in Deed, and According to the Truths that I Teach, which are Missing from the Pages of your Mutilated Bible. (See: *Second Chronicles 9:29 and Related Scriptures.*)

06-09 [_] Now, I Hear someone, who is like a Slender Workhorse, whinny: "O Peacock, I have been Eating mostly Raw Fruits and Vegetables for many Years, and have been Working Hard for all of my Life; and therefore, WHY would I need to Change my Diet, in Order to Prepare for a Fast?"

06-10 [_] Well, O Workhorse, if your Bowels are Working Good, and you are Feeling Good, there is no Good Reason for you to Change your Diet: because you will probably be able to Fast with ease. Therefore, you can simply begin your Extended Fast by taking a 3- to 4-day Fast, and then Flush Out your Bowels with Prune Juice, which is one of the most Laxative Fruit Juices there is on this Earth, IF it is Good Prune Juice. Moreover, after you Drink that 32-ounce Bottle of Prune Juice, you may follow it with a Quart or Liter of some Kind of Fresh Fruit Juice an Hour later — such as Fresh Orange Juice, Grapefruit Juice, Watermelon Juice, Carrot Juice, or whatever you Like; but, make Sure that you Drink Enough Prune Juice, in Order to FLUSH OUT your Bowels during ONE DAY, beginning early in the Morning, and never at Night: because you need as much Sleep as possible before you do such Flushing.

06-11 [_] However, it is a *Lack of Sleep* that usually Drives most People to Breaking their Fasts: because of the Poisons that have Accumulated within their Bowels. Therefore, it is not the End of the World, if you have to Break your Fast at Night; but, it is Wiser to do it early during the Morning Hours, around 6 A.M., even though no one has ever woke up Hungry, that I know of: because Sleep seems to Re-adjust the Mind and Body with Reality.

06-12 [_] However, in spite of that Information, there is another Preferred Option, if you have Access to Fresh Immature Coconut Water, or even Bottled Coconut Water without any Coconut Meat in it. Indeed, the Fresh Immature Coconut Water is so Laxative that 2 Quarts or 2 Liters will normally go right on through your Bowels within an Hour or less, and will not Cause any Bloating Up with Gases, even if you are an 80-year-old Constipated Senior Graduate of the Public School of Ignorant Fools, who never Mention the Importance of FASTING.

06-13 [_] Now, I Hear someone, who is like a Delicate Chicken, squawk: "O Peacock, I am already Skinny, and I have the 'runs' all of the Time: and therefore, what Good will it do for me to Fast?"

06-14 [_] Well, O Chicken, you might not Believe it; but, Fasting can Cure you of those "Runs," and even Cause your Body to gain Weight; but, only after you get RID of whatever it is that is Causing your Body to Reject everything that you Eat, which could be the Bad Recycled Sewage Water that you are Drinking. Therefore, be Sure to Fast until your Body Corrects itself, and do not Fear to get Skinnier: because your Weight will come back to Normal, or whatever is Right for you, considering what Kind of a Body that you have Inherited from your Parents. After all, if they were all Skinny, you can also Expect to be Equally as Skinny: because you Inherited their Genes; but, chances are that your Body has never Lost its Youthfulness, which is WHY that it Attempts to Eliminate all Unnatural Foods for you, even though you Insist on Eating such Foods: because it is your Tradition to do so. Therefore, you will have to Change your Diet, if you Sincerely Want to Change your Looks; but, be Aware that you do not make any Radical Changes without Fasting, first: because you could have WORMS, which are more or less Consuming whatever you Eat. Therefore, you should Fast until those Worms come Out of you, which you might have Contracted by Eating Unclean RAW Vegetables, or by coming into Contact with some Unclean Restroom. After all, there are probably a million Different "Bugs" that can Inflict People, and many of them are Beneficial; but, most of them are Detrimental, or Harmful to some Degree, which can Reduce our Lifespans if we come into Contact with them. However, a certain Sickness or Disease can often Straighten Out a Lost Soul, and bring that Soul to a State of

Confession and Truth that he or she might not otherwise Experience. Therefore, *"all things work together for Good, ..."* as it is written, for those Humble Honest People who are Called and Chosen for some Special Purpose within the Holy Kingdom, or the Government of God. (See *Romans 8:28, KJV.*) Therefore, you can Thank the Creator for whatever Ails you: because it probably keeps you more Humble and Honest; and therefore, it is an Improvement of your Spirit, which must also be brought to Perfection with your Body: because they are Together, as One.

06-15 [_] Now, I Hear someone, who is like a Cat, meow: "O Peacock, it seems that whenever I Eat Flesh of any Kind, I have a Typical Cat-like Nature, which is very Temperamental or Moody; and therefore, I am wondering if Fasting will Cure me of that Problem?" Well, O Cat, you can simply Change your Diet, and Prove to yourself that it is that Flesh that makes you Moody, which makes you like a Cat that Purrs one Minute, and the next Minute you could be ready to Scratch Out someone's Eyes!

06-16 [_] Now, I Hear someone, who is like an Elephant, snort: "O Peacock, I have a Close Friend, who Eats a LOT of Flesh; and therefore, he Sleeps for about 16 Hours each Day, and is still Feeling TIRED; but, I have not been Able to Persuade him to GIVE UP his Bad Eating Habits, even though I only need 3 or 4 Hours of Sleep each Night, plus 2 or 3 so-called 'Cat Naps': because I am a Strict Vegetarian. Moreover, he also Smokes a lot, when he does Wake Up. Therefore, what can we Do for him, who seems to be Related with a Lion?"

06-17 [_] Well, O Elephant, it seems to be Strange that someone who is like a Lion would be your Friend; but, I suppose that you have your Good Reasons. Nevertheless, your Concern for him is no Doubt Related with the Fact that you Love him: because of his Good Looks, his Artistic Abilities, or because of his Love for you, since it is obviously not a Sexual Attraction: because it is very Difficult to be Romantic with someone who Sleeps for most of the Day. Therefore, if he does not Want to Change his Diet, and Eat with you, there is not much that you can Do, in Order to Persuade him to Change his Ways, except to Fast and Pray for him, until both of you are Changed: because there is Power in the Act of Fasting and Praying, which can bring about Marvelous Things for certain People. Indeed, it might be that your Friend does not Want to Change his Diet; but, it might be that he would like to Overcome his Addiction to Nicotine, which he can do by Fasting and Praying, combined with certain Days of Eating Sweet Fruits.

06-18 [_] However, it is Dangerous for a One-sided Meat-eater to Eat lots of Fruits, either before or after Fasting: because it could BLOAT UP such a Person, and could even Kill him: because of the Gases that would be Formed within his Bowels. Therefore, such a Person should go on my Transition Diet of Coleslaw, Red Garden Beets, Cooked Green Leaves, Green Onion Tops, and Lettuce: because such Foods will not Cause him to Bloat Up nor Feel Uncomfortable, until he gets a Diarrhea. Moreover, after a Month on such a Strict Diet, your Friend will Feel much more Alive, and will probably Realize that there is much more to be Gained by Self-denial, than by Self-indulgence. After all, Life consists of much more than Feasting with Ravenous Lions, Laughing Hyenas, Jackals, Painted Highly-perfumed Skunks, Drunken Ducks, and Wild Dogs.

06-19 [_] Indeed, some Rebellious People take Great PRIDE in being One-sided Meat-eaters, who never Cross the Line nor Pollute themselves with Fruits nor Vegetables: because they

Vainly Imagine that they are Stronger than Vegetarians. However, the Great Apes are about 8 Times as Strong as an African Lion; and a Vegetarian Elephant is about 10 Times as Strong as a Meat-eating Dog, in proportion to their Weights. In other Words, if a Dog were as large as an Elephant, the Elephant would still be about 10 Times as Strong as that huge Dog: because there is something very Weakening about Eating Flesh, which provides very little Endurance, also. For Example, a Lion can produce a sudden Burst of Energy for a single Minute or so; but, the Wild Deers can run for Miles without getting Tired, and a Rhinoceros can run for 3 to 4 Days, nonstop, before he Wears Out: beCause of his Great Endurance on a Grasses-only Diet: because his Muscles are not Lugged Down by the Sticky Slime that is found in Digested and Assimilated Flesh.

06-20 [_] Moreover, an Elephant can easily Live for 80 Years; but, the Poor Lion does well to make it to 30 Years: because it Requires so much Energy for a Body to Eliminate that Flesh, which Causes the Lion to Sleep for 20 Hours per Day, while the Horse might Sleep for only 2 Hours per Day. Therefore, the LESS Flesh that any Person Consumes, the LESS Work his or her Organs will have to do, in Order to Eliminate the Waste Matter. Likewise, the LESS Sticky Greasy Fried Potatoes, Gummy White Breads, Gooey Cheeses, and Iced-creams that a Person Eats, the LESS Effort it will Require for his or her Body to Eliminate it.

06-21 [_] In Fact, a LIGHT Meat-eater might easily Outlive a HEAVY Bean and Bread Eater, if that Meat-eater also Eats lots of Greens: because the Body might more easily Handle it. Moreover, when you consider how that the Human Body is Basically just a PIPE SYSTEM, it only makes Good Sense to run Fruit Juices through those Pipes, as Opposed to Trying to run Cheeseburgers through them. Nevertheless, each Person must make his or her own Decisions about what to Eat: because we Adults are all Free to do so; and we will all have to Suffer for our Dietary Sins, IN AS MUCH AS we go to Extremes. Therefore, let each Person be Wise for him or herself: because, when it comes to Eating, we have to Bear our own Burdens, even if we do not like them: beCause, who else can Carry about such Blubber for us?

06-22 [_] Now, I Hear someone, who is like a Bear, growl: "O Offensive Peacock, in my Opinion, it makes little or no Difference what a Person Eats: because it will all go on through, sooner or later, if we do Enough Fasting. Therefore, there is no Need for anyone to Prepare for a Fast."

06-23 [_] Well, O Bear, just because you can get by with Eating just about anything, it does not Mean that other People can get by with it: because many People would be SICK, and Especially if they were to Eat some Old Rotten Flesh that some Hungry Bear has Stored in his Refrigerator for a Year or 2. Therefore, let each Person take Full Responsibility for his or her own Actions, and do whatever he or she Knows is Best: because, if anyone Suffers, it will be According to his or her own Decisions — not mine.

— Chapter 07 —

How LONG should a Person Fast?

07-01 [_] Well, once again, each Person must Judge his or her own Physical Condition, according to how he or she Feels, while Remembering the LAW of COMPENSATION, which is this: *"We all Reap whatever we Sow."* In other Words, if we have Eaten like Hogs, and have Accumulated 200 to 400 Pounds too much within our Bodies, we must Suffer for it while it is being Eliminated. Likewise, if we have Eaten a lot of Flesh, Eggs, Cheese, Candy, and other Super Sticky Stuff (SSS), we can Expect Fasting to be very Difficult: because the Body can hardly squeeze Out such Concentrated Slime, which is like thick Glue: because, when Flesh is Boiled Down, it forms GLUE from the Broth.

07-02 [_] Indeed, all Kinds of Broths from all Kinds of Flesh can be and has been made into Furniture Glue, Bookbinder's Glue, and all Kinds of GLUE: because it is very STICKY, which is also WHY it Sticks Inside of Human Bodies, CAUSING Various Kinds of Ailments, ranging from Common Colds, Flqz, Measles, Mumps, Chicken Pox, Arthritis, Rheumatism, Gout, and Kidney Stones to Gallstones, and so on: because, as in the Cases of Kidney Stones and Arthritis, the Glue STICKS Together with Limestone Deposits from Drinking or Eating Hard Water, which Crystallizes in the Joints, Kidneys, Bladder, or wherever it can Lodge.

07-03 [_] Moreover, when any Kind of Grain is BOILED DOWN, it forms a PASTE or STICKY SLIME, which is called MUCUS when it is Discharged from the Body in the Form of a so-called "COLD," which is nothing more than an *Accumulation* of Excess SLIME, or MUCUS, which the Body is Trying to Eliminate, or get Rid of by Means of the "Cold," which should be called a "Mucus Discharge." However, that Mucus does not always get Eliminated by Means of a Cold: because the Body loses its Ability to Discharge certain Super Sticky Filth. (NOTE: Even a Horse can "Catch a Cold," if you Feed to it too much Grain, such as too much Oats or Barley.)

07-04 [_] For Example, when the Mucus from Super Sticky Sugar, or Egg Whites, Lodges in an Eyeball, the Doctor calls it a Cataract, which is just an Accumulation of SLIME, which might consist of Slime from a hundred or more Different Kinds of Flesh, Grains, Candies, Eggs, or whatever such a Person has been Eating, which has Digested and Deposited itself in the Eyeball by Means of the Bloodstream, which Bloodstream is also Used by the Body, in Order to make Deposits of similar Slime, Fats, Oils, Mucus, Harmful Chemicals, and Poisons of Various Kinds throughout the entire Body, from Head to Toe: because there is no other Way for that Filth to get there, except by the Bloodstream, which is like the Highway that Carries all Kinds of Traffic with all Kinds of Cargo, including Healthy Vitamins, Minerals, Proteins, Sugars, Fats, and so on, which certain Organs of the Body are Supposed to SORT OUT, SEPARATE, and ELIMINATE whatever the Body does not Want or Need.

07-05 [_] Indeed, that Greasy Dandruff that People scratch off of their Scalps, after not taking a Bath for a few Days, must have Originally come from the Stomach, by Means of the Internal Pipe Systems, which begin at the Mouth in the Head, and ends up coming Out of the Mouth of the Anus. However, X-amount of that Food comes Out of the Pores of the Skin, as well as Out of the Nose, Throat, Eyes, Ears, and Urine: because all Openings of the Body are Wisely Used by the Body, in Order to Expel or get Rid of any Excess Waste Matter, even if the Body must Vomit it back Out of the Mouth from which it Entered: because the Body has its own Mind, you might say, and it always at least TRIES to Save itself from the Fool who Imagines that he or she is in Command of it, even if that Body must become PARALYZED, get LOCK JAW, go INSANE, or go into a COMA!

07-06 [_] In Fact, every Sickness and Disease that a Person gets is simply the Body's Way of making Compensations or Adjustments for the Bad Eating Habits of whomever is Supposedly in Command of such a Body, who Refuses to Listen to the Body's own Demands — one of which is to Stop Eating just as soon as a Person Feels Satisfied, whereby a very Small Amount of Sweet Fruits can Satisfy a Person's Appetite, and even "Spoil" a Ravenous Appetite!

07-07 [_] Therefore, as a Parent, do not Blame your Children for the Colds, Flqz, and Diseases that they get: because you are the one who is Feeding them all of those Mucus-forming Foods, including so-called "Healthy" Cereals for Breakfast, which are often half Sugar, which has been Highly Refined at Sugar Factories, which Sugar immediately enters into the Bloodstream: because the Body does not have to Process it: because it is already Highly Refined and Processed. Indeed, the Body would Normally have to Digest and Process any Kind of WHOLE Foods — such as Beans, Meats, and Potatoes; but, with Highly Refined Foods, there is no Need for Processing it, except to immediately ABSORB it into the System; and then Deal with it later on, whenever such a Person FASTS, gets SICK, or just STOPS EATING BREAKFAST, and gives to the Body a CHANCE to Eliminate it.

07-08 [_] In Fact, most Bodies of most Creatures have a small Chance to Eliminate some Waste Matter each Day, during the Night, while that Creature is Sleeping; but, certain Unenlightened People will actually get up during the Night, and EAT! Yes, their Stomachs are already Protruding with Excess Wastes, and yet they Feel HUNGRY — STARVED to Death, you might say, for whatever Leftovers are in the Refrigerator! But, the Truth is, they are only Tormented by the Excess Acids in their Stomachs, and by their LUSTS: because they have Allowed certain Longing Desires into their Minds, which can only be Eliminated by Self-denial, Self-discipline, and by FASTING and PRAYING.

07-09 [_] In Fact, they must get DESPERATE about Fasting, and REFUSE to even Think about Foods: because they are Overcome by it: because it has Control over them, rather than the other way around. Indeed, they might have to Clean OUT the Refrigerator of all Foods, and Post a large Sign on the Door of it, which reads:

07-10 [_] **"I am a Food Addict, who has been Overcome by my Lusts; and therefore, I Pray that God will Help me to DENY myself, before I go to Hell with the Irreverent LOUDMOUTH Sloth-gut Windbag Hole-in-his-Head, who needs a Wheelbarrow just to Pack his own Stomach around and throughout his House of Hate, who is a Good Example of someone that I do not Want to be Like."**

07-11 [ ] Now, after your Bowels have been FLUSHED OUT with Prune Juice, Grape Juice, Orange Juice, Immature Coconut Water, or even with Herbal Laxatives and Water, you can Fast with ease for at least 4 or 5 Days, before you will need another similar "Flush," at which Time you can easily Fast for another 5 to 6 Days; and then give to yourself another Flush with Juices; and then Fast for another 6 to 7 Days, and take another Flush, followed by another Fast of 7 to 10 Days on nothing but Pure Spring Water, followed by another Flush with Fruit Juices, followed by another Fast of 10 to 20 Days, or until your Tongue is CLEAN, like that of a little Baby, or like that of a Puppy, whose Tongue is PINK — not Coated with Thick Yellow Slime, or PLAQUE, like that of Poor Old Misses Irreverent LOUDMOUTH Sloth-gut Windbag Hole-in-her-Head, who says that "God does not Judge by the Inward Appearance of the Bowels; but, only by how much Makeup and Perfume that a Person uses, in Order to Camouflage the Truth, or Hide the Dietary Sins." †§

07-12 [ ] Yes, she Sincerely Believes that there is no such a Thing as a HOLY Person, who has a CLEAN Body and Mind: because, to her, even a Baby is UNHOLY, and will even go to Hell, if that Baby is not "SAVED" by a Water Baptism! That is, According to Misses LOUDMOUTH, even a Child must REPENT, by saying: "O Lord, I have been Thinking Evil, Vainly Imagining that I am going to go to Hell, if I do not Accept you as my Lord and Savior, even though I cannot Understand WHY that I would Need a Savior; but, I can See that Poor Old Misses Irreverent LOUDMOUTH Sloth-gut Windbag Hole-in-her-Head most certainly Needs a SAVIOR: because she cannot Resist Eating 10 Times more than she Needs for Nourishment, which is WHY that she Weighs 450 Pounds, and still INSISTS on COOKING! Yes, if any Person Needs to be SAVED, it is SHE who Preaches the False Doctrines of the Irreverent LOUDMOUTH Sloth-gut Windbag Hole-in-his-Head, who is Related to a Walrus, who Denies the Fact that there are Clean and Unclean People, who come in all Degrees of Cleanness and Uncleanness." §

07-13 [ ] Please notice the Stickiness of Fried Chickens, as you Eat them by using your Bare Fingers to hold the Piece of Chicken up to your Mouth; and also notice how much that Chicken STINKS, as you Smell of it, just before you Eat it; and Understand that no Wild Animal on this Earth will Eat anything, until it SMELLS of it, in Order to Discover whether or not it Smells GOOD or BAD; and if it Smells Bad, that Animal will not Eat it. Therefore, you and I will do Well to Accept a Lesson from Nature, and SMELL of our Foods before we Eat them. Yes, pull the Flesh off of the Bones with your Fingers, and Smell of it, FIRST, before you Decide to Eat something that STINKS to you like Unappetizing Raw Chicken GUTS!

— Chapter 08 —

How to BREAK a Fast

08-01 [_] Now, if you have Followed the Rules for Fasting thus far, you have Understood that each Body is UNIQUE, and must be Treated Individually: beCause there are always Exceptions to the RULES, which is WHY that they are called "RULES," instead of "LAWS." Indeed, *Laws are Unalterable,* like the so-called *"Law of Gravity,"* which is an Invisible Force that Attracts or Repels everything toward the Center of the Earth, according to its Weight or Mass; but, Rules are Flexible, like Yield Signs at Highways, where you can Look, STOP and/or Proceed.

08-02 [_] Therefore, each Person must make up his or her own PERSONAL Rules to some Degree concerning Fasting: because General Rules might not be Exactly Right for him or her. Nevertheless, as a General Rule, all Fasts should be Broken with LAXATIVE Foods, which are Foods that easily pass through the Bowels as Quickly as Possible, as Opposed to CONSTIPATING Foods — such as Sticky Gooey Peanut Butter, Cheese, Grease, Cow Butter, Flesh, White Gummy Bread, Candies, Potatoes, Beans, Cereals, Grains, Milk, Eggs, and even certain Kinds of Greens: because they Require too much Time to pass through the Bowels, causing the Body to REABSORB much or most of the Slime and Poisons that have been SQUEEZED or Excreted from the Body into the Bowels while Fasting.

08-03 [_] In other Words, when you do Decide to Break a Fast, you must have your Mind SET for one Primary Purpose, which is NOT to Feed yourself some "Good Nourishing Foods"; but, to SWEEP OUT your Bowels with as much Laxative Fruits or Juices as are Necessary, in Order to CLEAN OUT your Bowels of as much Slime and Poisons as Possible: because that will leave you Feeling Strong and Healthy and thus Happy, and especially IF you manage to Eliminate ALL of those Poisons that were previously making you Feel WEAK and Miserable.

08-04 [_] ***Moreover, the sooner that all such Filth is Removed from the Bowels, after Breaking a Fast, the Stronger and Better that you will Feel.*** Indeed, Healthy Bowels will Eliminate most of the Slime and Accumulated Filth within them within 10 to 15 Minutes, while Sluggish Bowels might Require as much as 6 Hours or more, Depending on how Constipated a Person is, or how Starved a Person is. After all, there comes a Point where a very Skinny Person's Body wants to Retain whatever Foods get into it; but, that is most likely NOT the Case for YOU: because you have not been nearly Starved to Death in some Nazi Concentration Camp: beCause the Allies (Great Britain, France, the United States of America, and Union of Soviet Socialist Republicans) have BOMBED the Railways and Bridges throughout Germany and Poland, and thus Cut Off your Food Supplies, and then Falsely Blamed your Starvation onto those Naughty Germans, who Historically Treated their Prisoners of Wars (POWs) Humanely, and so Humanely that only ONE American POW Died in a German Prison Camp, and it was not from Starvation; but, from one American Murdering another one. Therefore, let us Try to get the Record Straight, after Proving it in a Courtroom. Indeed, an Honest White Jew by the Name of Benjamin Freedman has Thoroughly Explained it on a YouTube Video for whomever might Want to Learn the Whole Truth about it. *"Seek, and you shall Find."* †‡

08-05 [_] Furthermore, after using Fruit Juices, in Order to Break a certain Number of Fasts, the Body will get Used to those Juices, and will not have such a Positive Reaction to Drinking them. Indeed, I, for Example, must Drink at least 2 whole 32-ounce Bottles of Prune Juice, plus a half gallon of Orange Juice, just to get a Bowel Movement: because of doing so much Fasting and Flushing. In Fact, if I do not Fast for at least one Week, on nothing but Water, and then Drink a LOT of Juice, it will all just Reabsorb into my System, and it will make me Feel very Weak and Poisoned, which is no Good. Therefore, I must also Follow the Rules.

08-06 [_] Moreover, if I were to Fast for one whole Month, with Periodical Flushes, and then, just after Flushing during a Friday, for Example, were to Attempt to get another Flush during the following Sunday or Monday, I might even Kill myself by such Bad Actions, or at least Thoroughly Poison myself, and thus Waste that Time, altogether. Therefore, if you are going to Fast, you have to lay aside all of your Worldly Ambitions and make up your Mind that you are going to Faithfully Follow the RULES as Closely as Possible, and **never Attempt to Flush Out your Bowels within any less than 4 Whole Days after the Previous Flush.**

08-07 [_] Now, I Hear someone, who is like a Confused Sheep of the Good Shepherd, bleat: "O Peacock, are you saying that it is not SAFE for us to Fast, unless we FLUSH OUT our Bowels after each Fast? For Example, I have an Aunt Wretched, who Fasts every Moonday and Marsday: because she Eats too much on Saturnday and Sunday: because it is her Tradition to do so. Indeed, she Knows that she is going to Fast on Moonday, and therefore she Overeats on Sunday. Moreover, her Body seems to Retain whatever she Eats on Sunday, until she Breaks her Fast on Mercuryday or Weddingday, which she Breaks by Eating Whole Wheat Bread: because she says that 'if it was good enough for the Apostle Paul, it is good enough for me.' (See *Acts 27, KJV.*) And she also points out the Fact that Jesus Fed the Multitudes with Whole Grain Bread and Fishes, after they had not Eaten for 3 Days. (See *Matthew 14; Mark 6; Luke 9; John 6; and Matthew 15:32.*) Therefore, according to my Aunt Wretched, the only Proper Food for a Person to Break a Fast on, is *Biblical* BREAD and FISHES, even though she does Confess that it might Help to Eat some Fresh Fruits, or at least squeeze out some Lemon Juice on her Bread: because that Helps to break down some of the Sticky Slime in it. Likewise, it also Helps those Fishes to Digest, and somewhat Neutralize the Stickiness of them. Therefore, is it OKAY for us to Break our Fasts on such a Diet as that?"

08-08 [_] Well, O Sheep, it seems to be rather Strange that you would have any Desire to Eat Fishes; but, if you Insist, you can do it, and probably will do it, in spite of whatever I might have to say about it: because you have Confidence in what your Aunt Wretched is doing. However, she only gets by with such an Act beCause of the Fact that she only Fasts for 2 Days; and therefore, she does not really get much of an Elimination of Filth and Poisons within such a Short Time: because her Bowels can barely get Rid of the Previous Meals during Sunday, before they are Overloaded with some more Fishes and Bread on Wednesday. Therefore, she is only Helping to Relieve herself of the Excess Food that she Ate during Sunday, which does Help her to some Degree; but, it will never Replace a TRUE Fast, which must be carried out for as long as it Requires, in Order for the Body to Eliminate ALL of the Accumulated Filth that is Lodged within it, which might Require as much as 7 Years of Self-discipline, as you can read in a Quotation within: **"HOW to Become a HOLY Man!" (40 Good Reasons WHY People Should FAST and PRAY!) By The Worldwide People's Revolution!®** Book 045.

08-09 [_] Indeed, many Americans will have to Abstain from Eating any Flesh, Eggs, Cheeses, White Breads, Nuts, Iced-creams, Cookies, Candies, and all such Super Sticky Stuff (SSS) for perhaps 10 to 20 Years, just to Regain their Youthfulness, unless they take up Fasting and Praying According to these Proper RULES for FASTING, which can Reduce that Time to 2 to 3 Years, if they Exercise much Self-discipline, and do not Eat too much at any Meal between Fasts and Flushes.

08-10 [_] **However, when you are Breaking a Fast, you do not Dare MINCE on a few Dates, Figs, Raisins, or some other Concentrated Fruit: beCause you MUST Consume Enough Foods to CAUSE a Good Bowel Movement, right away, followed by several Good Bowel Movements within that same Day. Otherwise, a certain Amount of the Poisons and Filth, which were Squeezed into your Bowels while Fasting, will be REABSORBED back into your System, and that will POISON you and WEAKEN you, and perhaps even Discourage you from Fasting, which has Happened to many Unbelievers and Disobedient BRATS, who almost never Want to Blame themselves for anything that has gone WRong!**

08-11 [_] Moreover, if you Eat Fruits while Breaking a Fast, you can also BLOAT UP from GASES: because, when Fruits are MIXED with the Slime of Meats, Eggs, Cheeses, and other similar Matter, it will Naturally FERMENT, even as it would do within a Pot on the Stove at 98 degrees Fahrenheit, or 36.66 °C. In Fact, just for the FUN of it, you can Pretend that you are an Honest Scientist, who can Chew Up and Spit Out your Thanksgiving Dinner into a Cooking Pot, or whatever Foods that you Imagine are Good for you to Break a Fast on, and Scientifically Examine it within a Laboratory for Gases and Acids during the next 24 Hours, while keeping it Warm on the Stove; and then Ask yourself if such a Deadly Mixture of Foods could possibly be GOOD for you to Eat, considering the Fact that your Bowels must SORT OUT whatever you put into them, and keep you Alive at the same Time? After all, when a Person VOMITS, he or she gets a Realistic Look, Smell, Taste, and Feel of whatever he or she Imagines is Good for him or her to Eat, which is one of the most Unpleasant Experiences of his or her Life, until AFTER all of the Poisons have been Vomited OUT; and then it is a Great Relief to get Rid of them.

08-12 [_] Likewise, when such a Person gets a Diarrhea, he or she gets a Firsthand Experience of the Horrible Mixtures of FILTH that have been Lodged within his or her Bowels, which no Wild Animal on this Earth Experiences: because they do not Eat a million Combinations of Capitalist Concoctions, much less Charge anyone Money for Preparing such Concoctions for the Purpose of bringing about Sicknesses, Diseases, and Deaths. Indeed, LIFE, itself, could not possibly come from any such Concoctions, even if certain Deceived Women think so; and, as for that Fat Chef, whose Protruding Stomach Testifies against him, he can Cheerfully Agree with me that Life would be a lot less Burdensome if there were NO Cooking, NO Dishwashing, NO Greasy Walls to Clean, NO Greasy Clothes to Wash, NO Sicknesses, nor any Diseases. Yes, he can Agree with me that I have Escaped many Sicknesses, just by AVOIDING all such Feasts for Fools.

08-13 [_] However, from Poor Beggars to Rich Queens and Royal Kings, there is nothing so Inviting as a Sumptuous Meal of Dog Food or Hog Slop, if it is put Together in the Right Order by Deceptions and Lies, being Spiced with certain Prayers of Thanksgiving, and Spread Out on the Tables of Lust and Greed, where it is Consumed by Ignorant Idiots and Misguided Fools, who Vainly Imagine that they will Die and go to Heaven, where the Holy Angels will have much Better Banquets on Tables that are Miles Long, being Covered with all Kinds of DRIED Cow's PUSS, Puddings, CAKES, Pies, and Globs of SLIME from which they will FEAST for ever and ever with Eternal BLISS: beCause their Bodies will be Able to Handle it, being made in the Image of GOD, who Naturally Feasts at such a Long Table, every Day: beCause it is the Glory of both God and Man to make Fools of themselves at least once a Week, if not every Day.

08-14 [_] In Fact, According to their Religion, there is only ONE Forbidden Food, and that is the Sweet Juicy Fruit from the Tree of the Knowledge of All that is Good and Evil, which Fruit is Supposedly an APPLE! {NOTE: The Fruit from that Tree Represented all Forbidden Foods.} However, what makes a Better Drink than Good Apple Cider, which has been Spiced with just enough Vodka to make Poor Old Aunt Wretched Confess that she has a long, LONG Ways to go, before she will be Able to Compete with Poor Old Uncle Miserable, when it comes to Inventing Self-inflicted Punishments? However, when Uncle Miserable gets Together with Aunt Wretched, and both of them set Ultraistic Goals, which only Rich People could ever Afford, such Dreams become American Nightmares, like we now have, wherein X-amount of People are in such a Hellish Condition, that they cannot See any Way Out, except to commit Suicide!

08-15 [_] However, all such People could Change their Diets, and Live mostly on Fruits and Vegetables, if they could Afford them, now that they have Departed from the Land that might Feed and Clothe them. Moreover, they could also do a certain Amount of Fasting during Weekends, Holidays, and Vacations, if they had a LOT of Willpower. Nevertheless, such Fasts will only Frustrate the Person who Attempts to do them: because the Goal is Holiness of Mind, Spirit and Body; and that is Impossible without a Full-time Commitment, which will Require a New Jerusalem, where People can Help each other to Fast, while also Providing much of their own Foods; but, at least they will not have to be Tormented by all of the Problems that Face the Citiots, who Allow People who are like Lions and Wolves to come in among them — such as that Sniper who Terrorized Washington, D.C., Years Ago, which needs to be Terrorized by something: because it is the Headquarters for Chief Criminals in **"The Divided States of United Lies!" (The so-called "United States of North America" in Disguise!)** Book 058. {See also: **"Poverty Hunger Riots Strikes Brutalities Election Deceptions and Civil Wars!" (The High Price that we Earthlings have Paid for Leaving the Good Land!) By The Worldwide People's Revolution!® Book 014.**}

08-16 [_] Yes, the District of Corruption, in Washington, is the Headquarters for the Chief Criminals, beginning with the President of Political Rabbits, who FROWNS on SEPARATION and SEGREGATION, as if the Kingdom of God will have both Saints and Sinners in the same City of Confusion, seeing that Sinners like to SIN, and Saints like to FAST. Indeed, the Highest Calling of a Sinner is to get Drunk and go to Bed with some Pretty Highly-perfumed Painted SKUNK; but, the Highest Calling of a Saint is to be like Jesus Christ, who is the King of his own World, who has no Interest in Vain Sensual Pleasures: beCause his Mind is on Higher Goals and Spiritual Subjects. Nevertheless, that is not to say that he does not Enjoy Eating Good Sweet Fruits: because that is Natural and Good, just as long as it is within the Bounds of Reason and Moderation. After all, even Sweet Fruits can be Mixed Together with all Kinds of Nuts, and made into Sensual Dishes for Lustful People, who can Overeat on those Tasty Dishes. Nevertheless, Jesus said, *"There is only Need for one Thing, which is Holiness of Mind, Spirit, and Body; and Mary has Chosen that more Blest Part, which has a Better Reward in the End.''* See *Luke 10:38—42, NMV.*

08-17 [_] I Recommend that each Person should first Drink Fruit Juices when Breaking a Fast, in Order to get the Bowels Working, followed by Fresh Fruits, if possible, which are not Poisoned with Sprays of any Kinds, nor even Grown by the Use of Harmful Chemicals and Poisons. And after that, a Person should pay Strict Attention to the next Chapter.

08-18 [_] However, the Ideal Fasting Plan is to FLUSH OUT your Bowels with Immature Coconut Water, and then Continue on Fasting for as long as you can stand it, on a Limited Amount of Pure Water; and then Repeat the Coconut Water Flush, until at last you are FREE! Yes, it might Require 80 Days or more to Accomplish it, if you are Old. Moreover, you should also mix the Juice of a few Fresh Ripe Limes with the Gallon of Coconut Water, which will Help to Loosen Up and Remove the Worst of Accumulated Filth. Be Sure to Brush your Teeth after it.

— Chapter 09 —

What to EAT after Breaking a Fast

09-01 [_] This is the Territory that most People get Lost in: because, while Fasting, they have been Lusting after all Kinds of "Goodies," which they Plan on Eating, just as soon as Possible: beCause their Lusts have been Craving all such Things. Therefore, being Hungry to some Degree, they are apt to Plunge Headlong to the Bottom of the Pit of Lusts, if they are not Careful: because, after Fasting for just a few Days, almost every Thing in a Kitchen will Smell Appetizing, and Taste even more Appetizing: because of all of the Spices and Aromas in the Process of Cooking, itself.

09-02 [_] Indeed, the Aromas of Baked Breads, Cakes, Cookies, Candies, and even Barbecued Flesh can be Overwhelming to any Hungry Soul, who is also Skinny and Ready to EAT! However, if such a Person is not Careful, he or she could easily Undo anything that was Gained by Fasting: because of Eating Foods that are not Laxative Enough, or because of Reabsorbing Old Poisonous Slime because of Eating only a Small Amount of Food. Therefore, if you are in a Famine Situation, and you do not have Enough Food, in Order to Break a Fast PROPERLY, you are better off to Resist the Temptation to Break the Fast, until you can get some Help.

09-03 [_] After all, there is usually something left to Eat, which other People "turn up their Noses at," as they say: because one of the Best Foods is Fresh Garden Greens, which you can also Grow, if you have some Seeds, Topsoil, Sunlight and Water. Yes, such Greens will Grow while you are Fasting, except during Winter Months in Extreme Climates; and some Greens will even Grow during the Winter — such as Kale and Collards, which will Grow even more with some Protection from a Greenhouse of some Kind, if you can Afford to Buy one, and have some Place to put it. Most People do not: because they are Extremely Poor — Thanks to Capitalism.

09-04 [_] Moreover, Swiss Chard can be Grown the Year around in the South, and is therefore quite Reliable, if you have Water; and only a few Plants will Sustain you through a Famine, if your Topsoil is Rich Enough. In other Words, you will not need Acres of Swiss Chard, Kale, nor Collards; but, you will need about 100 Plants per Adult Person. Furthermore, it will also Help to have a Variety of Greens, including Green Onions, Green Garlic, and Broccoli, which can be Grown in a Small Space. For Example, a Broccoli Plant can have as many as 200 Heads on just ONE Plant; and therefore, just 2 or 3 such Plants will keep you from Starving to Death; and especially if you have some Honey or Raisins, in order to Supplement your Diet, which can be Stored for many Years in a Cool Consistent Climate, and still be Good to Eat, if the Raisins are Vacuum-packed. Nevertheless, if everyone is in a Great Famine, and there is nothing to Eat, you are at the Mercy of Angels, who can Feed you, and who will Feed you, if they Discover that you are Worthy of it. Otherwise, it is a Good Idea to have LOTS of Survival Foods Canned up and ready to Eat when you Need them, including Bottled Fruit Juices, and not Sugar Water Drinks. Frozen Nuts also keep well for many Years, if the Temperature is Consistent, and if the Nuts are Vacuum-packed in Canning Jars. Raw Sunflower Seeds are also quite Nutritious and Satisfying.

09-05 [_] Now, I Hear someone, who is like a Crow, caw: "O Peacock, are you Suggesting that none of those Poor African Children, who are Starving to Death, are WORTHY of the Assistance of Holy Angels: because they are such Great Sinners? Surely, you must have been reading your *Bible* with a Closed Mind! After all, IF there is a God, he must be a God of JUSTICE; and therefore, any one of those little African Children is Equally as Qualified for the Assistance of Angels as you or anyone else is." †

09-06 [_] Well, O Crow, you need to read your *Bible,* once again: because you Missed the Message! Indeed, God IS a God of Justice, as you say; and therefore, it would be Unjust for him to Bless those Unholy Children with the same Gifts and Blessings that he Blesses his Holy Children with, who Call on him for Help; and as for those little Children who are Innocent and Ignorant, God Allows them to Die, in Order to bring us to Judgment for Allowing it: because we have the Responsibility of Caring for other Helpless People; and we also have all Kinds of Opportunities to do Good for them; but, we would rather Appropriate Trillions of Dollars for War Machines, War Games, and Lunar Explorations. Indeed, we Americans spend a hundred times more Money on SPORTS and Perfumes, than we do on Welfare for such Poor Deprived Souls in Africa: because we Judge that Sports and Perfumes are more Important.

09-07 [_] Moreover, we Americans spend or Waste more than 4 Trillion Dollars per Year on Medical Care, as a Result of Eating 10 times more than we Need! After all, we Sincerely Care for our GOOD HEALTH, which Begins with 3 Square Meals per Day, followed by several Hours of sitting in front of a TV: because we have not Discovered Gardening, or some Hobby that might otherwise keep us Occupied and Exercised.

09-08 [_] Nevertheless, God is only Interested in Saving certain Souls Alive: because the other Souls are Good Examples for what we do not Want to be Living Like — such as the Ignorant Fools in Africa, who do not have Reliable Sources of Foods, who do not even have Mango Trees, Cherimoyas, Coconuts, Bananas, Limes, nor Greens in their Gardens; but, worse than that, they do not even have large Cisterns for Water Storage: because it has never crossed their Weak Minds that such Cisterns are Needed, or else they are just too Poor to Afford to Build them, being somewhat like Americans, who would rather spend their Money on SPORTS, Drugs,

Alcohol, Cigarettes, Candies, Cokes, or at least on some MEAT: because, to them, those Things are much more Important than Cisterns full of Water. ‡

09-09 [_] Indeed, if they did get some extra Money, they would have to spend it on Cars, Army Vehicles, Airplanes, or at least on Hospitals, Drugs and Medical Doctors. However, what is Needed are those **"GLORIOUS Swanky Hotels Castles and Fortresses!" (Beautiful Planned City States for WISE Intelligent Well-Educated People with Common Sense and Good Understanding!) By The Worldwide People's Revolution!®** Book 019. Yes, all such City States are Designed to Protect the People from Wild Animals, while at the same Time provide them with Proper Water and Food Storage Facilities.

09-10 [_] Howbeit, if you think that those Poor Africans are in Trouble, you might want to Consider what an Awful Condition that most Americans will be in when the Rain STOPS: because Americans are not Used to Living on next to nothing. And oh what Great Regrets that Americans will have, when there is nothing to Eat nor Drink, and those Americans Remember the BILLIONS of Barrels of Gas and Oil that they have Wasted, just running to Work and back Home again, with nothing to Show for it, except Pollution, Acid Rains, Climate Changes, Accidents, Mangled Bodies, Junkyards, Empty Gas Tanks, and Great REGRETS! Indeed, we could have had Profitable and Secure Swanky Fortresses built for all of us with less Energy, and been Prepared for the Worst Conditions; but, instead, we Trusted that Wicked Anti-Christ FALSE Cover-up Federal Government in Washington, who had about as much Love for us, as they have for Fasting, which is ZILCH! Nevertheless, the Parade to Hell must go on, until we Learn our Lessons by one Means or another: because God has Determined to bring it to a Dramatic Catastrophic END.

09-11 [_] Now, I Hear someone, who is like a Frog, croak: "O Peacock, there will always be Sufficient Water for us to Drink: because we can Distill the Ocean Water, if it is Necessary for Survival; and we can Transport that Water to any Place in the World, even if it is in the Heartland of Africa: because all of the People in our Churches have Enough Love for them to do it. Yes, I just Heard a Report, last Week, which was telling how that we have had Compassion on those millions of People in Malawi, who have not had Rainwater in Sufficient Quantities within 3 Years, who are Barely Hanging on, who are Eating Dried Tree Leaves and Roots, just to Survive — that is, until we Christians Delivered a Trainload of Water and Foods for them on Imaginary Railroad Tracks, which Leap Over the Sand Dunes and Canyons — that is, just after they pass by hundreds of Gambling Casinos, Rich People's Hotels, and Theme Parks in South Africa." †§‡§§

09-12 [_] Well, O Frog, just one Cow Drinks about 10 to 50 gallons of Water per Day, depending on the Temperature, in Order to Produce 1 to 10 gallons of Milk per Day; and she also Eats a 100-pound Bale of Hay, plus 2 or 3 gallons of Grains; and therefore, the Space that is used for Growing Food for a Cow, could be used for Growing Foods for People; and the Water that she Drinks could be used for Watering Plants; but, in Africa, it is more Important for them to take Care of their Cattle, than themselves — that is, until a Famine comes, and then they Eat their Cattle; but, after 3 or 4 Years, most of their Cattle are also gone: because the Water runs Out, and the Food for Cattle also runs Out; and then those People are Forced to FAST, even though they would rather Eat. Likewise, Americans are likely to Face the same Problems, if they do not Wake Up and Realize what is more Important — Survival or Perfumes. But, why should I Care, since almost no one Listen to me?"

09-13 [_] If the Food is Available, I Recommend that you Eat nothing but Fresh RAW Sweet Juicy RIPE Unpoisoned Fruits for at least a whole Week after Fasting and Flushing, which have been Grown by **"The LUSCIOUS All-Mineral Organic Method of Gardening!" (HOW to Grow DELICIOUS Satisfying Foods for Potential Kingz and Kweenz in Swanky PALACES!) By The Worldwide People's Revolution!®** Book 021. However, the Possibility of that Happening is almost ZILCH: beCause of not having Swanky Fortresses to Live in. Therefore, you will just have to do the Best that you can with whatever you have to Work with.

09-14 [_] Check out your Local Health Food Stores, Farmers' Markets, and Naaberz' Gardens. Be Aware that Chemicals and Poisons will Wreck your Nerves, and Worrying about the Foods that you are Eating will Wreck your Nerves Worse than Eating Standard Chemically-grown Fruits and Vegetables; and not having Enough Money to Buy Good Wholesome Fruits and Vegetables could Cause you to CRASH, get Divorced, or whatever. Therefore, you can now Understand the "Back-to-the-Land Movement," during the 1960's and 70's. However, before you Attempt to do that, you should Study: **"The IDEAL Place to Live!" (HOW to Discover the Ideal Place to Live!) By The Worldwide People's Revolution!®** Book 069.

— Chapter 10 —

What should a Person Do while Fasting?

10-01 [_] Well, first of all, it is not a Time to Attempt to Work: because Working will also Work Up an Appetite to Eat, and then you will have to Eat. Otherwise, you will get Weak and Run Down. Therefore, it is Wise to just REST in Bed, and Understand that you are now lying on Nature's Operating Table, you might say, Patiently Waiting for Nature to do its Good Work within you, which is a very Slow but Sure Work.

10-02 [_] Indeed, while Resting, you can Listen to Recordings by the Peacock, who has Recorded most of his 350+ Inspired Books. And, other than that, you must take a Daily Shower, which will give to you some Exercise; and, if you Feel like it, you can go for a Short Walk in a Flower Garden; but, do not Attempt to Fulfill any Worldly Ambitions: because they will Surely Overcome you. Yes, many a Man has been Humiliated and Seduced by his own Ambitions: because it is Impossible to Serve 2 Masters at the same Time. (See *Matthew 6:16—34, NMV.*)

10-03 [_] As for myself, I spend most of my Time READING while Fasting. Otherwise, I Watch Interesting TV Programs, News Reports, C-SPAN, and Nature Programs. Other than that, I Pray and Meditate on the *Scriptures.*

— Chapter 11 —

Why do Muscles Twitch while Fasting?

11-01 [_] Well, the Fact is that Muscles can Twitch at any Time; but, while Fasting, the Twitching seems to Intensify, and thus becomes more Noticeable: because the Body is making an Effort to LOOSEN UP and SHAKE OUT any Unwanted Slime that might be Lodged within the Muscles, Organs, or Skin, including the Eyelids.

11-02 [_] Therefore, just be Patient, and the Twitching will soon Stop: because the Body will Accomplish its Goal, if you give to it a Chance.

11-03 [_] Moreover, you can Comfort yourself by Realizing that your Body is in Fact doing its Work to Eliminate certain Wastes. Remember that many People TWITCH for many Years: beCause of NOT Fasting, which is the only Sure Cure for that Problem, such as Twitching Eyelids.

— Chapter 12 —

Why are People PALE while Fasting?

12-01 [_] Well, if a Person has been Eating Cheese and Drinking Milk during the Past, such PALE-colored Foods will be Intensified in the Bloodstream during the Process of Elimination: because they are Super Sticky Foods, which can Lodge within the Body for Decades, or ever since Childhood. Moreover, the Blood is more Concentrated in the Central Organs, where it is used Wisely by the Body, in order to Try to Clean House in those Organs.

12-02 [_] Therefore, there is less Blood on the Surface of the Body: because it is not Needed there. Likewise, there is also less Blood for the Head, Hands, and Feet, which can make them Colder than normal.

12-03 [_] Moreover, because of the Paleness of the Skin, it lets other People know that you are "Sickly," which is Beneficial: because they are more apt to have Compassion for you, and even Voluntarily Help you. Therefore, when People Mock you for being Pale while Fasting, just Smile at them, and keep Silent: because that is your Strength.

12-04 [_] Yes, Hold your Peace within you, and Understand that they apparently do NOT Understand. Nevertheless, if they Insist on Learning WHY, you can Refer them to: **"HOW to Become a HOLY Man!" (40 Good Reasons WHY People Should FAST and PRAY!) By**

The Worldwide People's Revolution!® Book 045. However, be Aware that Truths will Cause a Division among you: beCause X-amount of People will Believe, while X-amount will not, who will Oppose you, and perhaps Ridicule and Mock you, even as they did for Jesus and his Disciples. Therefore, Moses, Elijah, John the Baptist, Jesus and Paul went into the Wilderness to do their Fasting and Praying, whereby they could be left alone. Yes, even Domesticated Dogs have been known to do the same Thing when they get Sick or Badly Wounded, who usually emerge in Good Health a Month or so later.

— Chapter 13 —

Why do People get DIZZY while Fasting?

13-01 [_] Well, once again, it is a Lack of Blood Pressure: because you are not Eating, which Means that less Blood is getting to the Brains, which Causes Dizziness, and Especially when you rise up Quickly, which seems to Rob what little Blood is getting to the Brains.

13-02 [_] Moreover, for that same Reason, the Brains can Malfunction, even while Resting in Bed: because of a Lack of Oxygen in the Blood and Brains. Therefore, before you get up, Remember to get up SLOWLY, and Breathe Deeply; and try to Increase the Amount of Oxygen in your Blood by DEEP Breathing for several Minutes before getting Up on your Feet.

13-03 [_] However, you do not Want to Overdo it on the Breathing: because that, alone, will Cause some People to get Dizzy. Therefore, sit up slowly, and roll out of Bed slowly: because you could possibly Faint after Standing Up too Quickly.

13-04 [_] However, in an Emergency, you might have to move Quickly, just to get to the Toilet, for which you should also have Plans for sitting down rather Quickly, within 2 Seconds or so, before you have Time to Faint or Collapse, which is WHY it is Important to have the Bed near to the Toilet, or the Portable Toilet near to the Bed when you are Breaking a Fast.

13-05 [_] Nevertheless, you will not Normally have such Problems, if you just Practice rising up SLOWLY, and try to hang onto something, if you are Old and Unstable. Otherwise, you might fall down and Crack your Skull Open, which will no Doubt Revise your Thinking in a Positive Way, and might even Discourage you from Fasting, all alone, as an Independent Jackass, when you Need some Help. Therefore, be Humble and Honest about it, before you are Hospitalized.

13-06 [_] Otherwise, you might become Discouraged with Fasting, altogether, which could Prove to be very Bad: because Fasting is your only Sure Cure for what Ails you. Therefore, Follow the Rules, and you will do Well. Indeed, as a First Resort, you should Commit yourself to a Swanky Fasting Sanitarium, where Professional People can Assist you, which you can Find at ALL of those **"GLORIOUS Swanky Hotels Castles and Fortresses!" (Beautiful Planned City States for WISE Intelligent Well-Educated People with Common Sense and Good Understanding!) By The Worldwide People's Revolution!®** Book 019.

— Chapter 14 —

What about Holding Conversations while Fasting?

14-01 [_] Well, most People do not Know it; but, those Conversations are often the Sources of their Greatest Weaknesses, whereby they give in to Drinking and Eating: because of Social Concerns, and because of not Wanting to be Left Out of the Popular Crowd. Indeed, you might have to Isolate yourself somewhere in the Wilderness, just to get Away from other People, who will be Tempting you to EAT, or to at least have a little DRINK of some Fruit Juice, or a Beer: because they Fear that you are "Wasting Away."

14-02 [_] Yes, they have seen Old People who not only Wasted Away; but, they also DIED: beCause they Insisted on Eating some Iced-cream, or at least Sucked on some Candy, which more or less SMOTHERED them to Death: because their Lungs filled up with SLIME that came from such Foods.

14-03 [_] Indeed, a Common Means of Death is by Pneumonia, which is Slime that is Stuck in the Lungs, which cannot easily be Coughed Out.

14-04 [_] However, if a Body is Working Correctly, it will Naturally Eliminate any Excess Slime or Mucus; and therefore, such a Person would not Suffocate to Death on his or her own Slime, even if he or she Contracted Pneumonia: because Fasting would quickly Remedy the Situation.

14-05 [_] Moreover, when a Sick Person Attempts to Speak, when he or she should keep Silent, it Upsets the entire Body, Causing a Mucus Discharge into the whole System, which often Causes a Person to COUGH UP Mucus, being somewhat like the Mucus Discharge that most People Experience after Eating a Meal, which Mucus should be Spit Out: because the Body is Trying to get Rid of it.

14-06 [_] Likewise, most People have Mucus in their Throats and Noses during the Morning, when they first get up, which should also be Spit Out; but, some People Swallow it and thus Recycle it for some Later Date with Doctor Death.

14-07 [_] However, after several Weeks of Fasting, all such Mucus Discharges will simply STOP, and you will at last Forget that you ever had them — that is, until you Eat some more Mucus-forming Foods, such as Grains, Dairy Products, Flesh, Candies, Potatoes, and Especially French-fried Potatoes, which are often Served on Dinner Plates for Victims of Capitalism, who have no Idea what they are Consuming at the Expense of their Lives.

14-08 [_] Moreover, if your Body is full of such Slime, you will also continue to have Mucus Discharges, in spite of Eating nothing but Fruits and Green Leaves: because such Mucus is Stored Up as Concentrated Glue, which slowly Loosens Up, Dissolves, and comes Out as a "Cold," if one does not Fast: because the Acids in the Fruits help to Dissolve such Sticky Slime, and Especially if you are Eating Citrus Fruits, which should be Juiced: because the White Parts of the Citrus Fruits are very Sticky, and are not at all Laxative, and the other Parts are Indigestible.

14-09 [_] **WARNING: Citrus Juice from Unripe Fruits is Guaranteed to RUIN your Precious Teeth: beCause of the Strong Acids. Therefore, be Sure to Rinse your Mouth Out with Clean Water, and Brush your Teeth Immediately after Drinking Citrus Juices in any Form;** *and follow that Cleansing with some Fresh Carrot Juice, if Possible, which you should swish around in your Mouth, which will somewhat Sooth your Teeth considerably more than just Pure Water.*

14-10 [_] Also, Drink any Citrus Juice through a **Straw,** so as to Help keep the Juice Off of your Teeth. And that also includes Drinking Immature Coconut Water with Lime Juice in it.

14-11 [_] Moreover, you must be Careful to not Eat too many Citrus Fruits, lest you should Loosen Up too much Mucus at one Time, and thus Poison your whole System: because of Overloading it with too much Mucus, which your Body cannot easily Eliminate, which could Cause certain Organs to FAIL!

14-12 [_] Therefore, it is Wise to Change your Diet SLOWLY and PERSISTENTLY, in Order to Succeed with your Cleansing Regime. Meanwhile, you might look Terrible to your Friends and Naaberz, which is all the more Reason why that you should keep SILENT and Maintain your PEACE of Mind. *"Finally, Brothers, whatsoever Things are Pure, whatsoever Things are Lovely, whatsoever Things are Honest, whatsoever Things are Pleasant, whatsoever Things can be Proven to be True, whatsoever Things Present Reasonable Solutions, and whatsoever Things are of a Good Report, Try to Think about those Things: because nothing is Gained by Thinking about Evil Things. Therefore, Set your Minds on All that is GOOD."* — NMV.

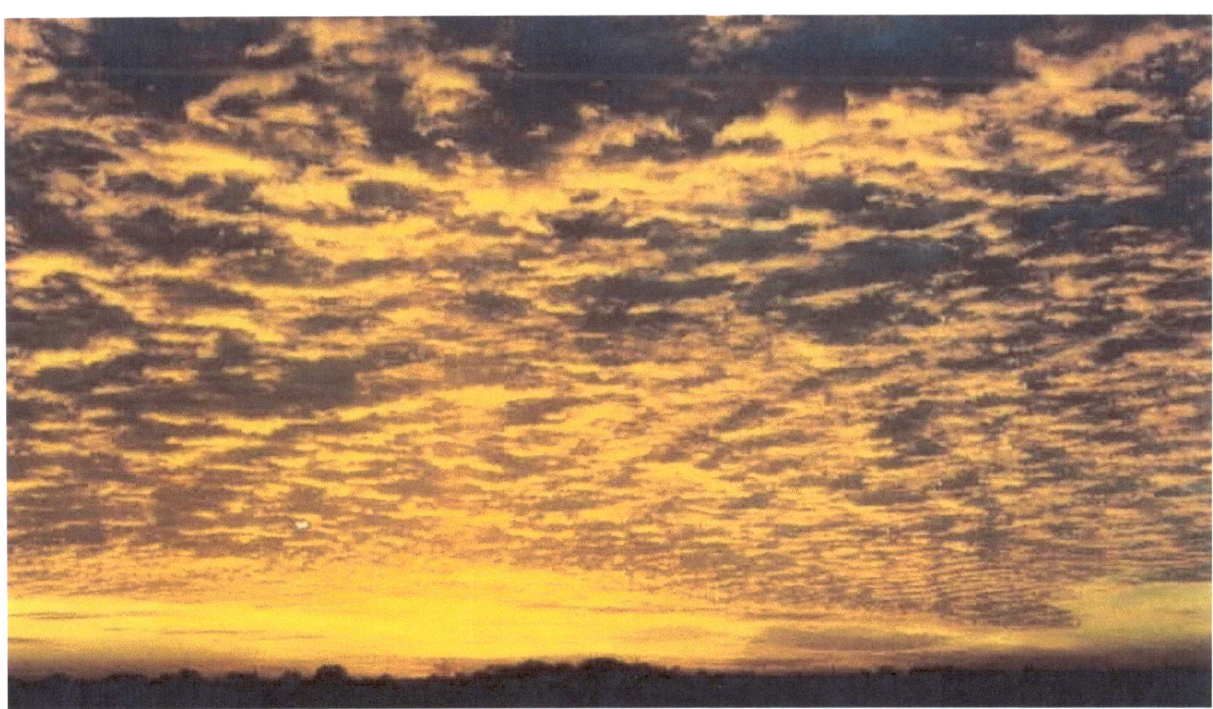

— Chapter 15 —

What about having SEX while Fasting?

15-01 [_] Well, if you cannot Resist the Temptation, having Sex will probably not Kill you; but, it will Weaken you to some Degree, unless you have not had Sex for a Long Time: because Sexual Fluids seem to be Nourishing to the Body; and having too much Sex seems to Drain a Person's Nerves of Vitality and Life, itself, which is WHY some Animals DIE after having Sex, such as Salmon. Therefore, while you are Denying yourself of Foods, Smoke, Drugs, Alcohol, and Vain Pleasures, you might as well be Denying yourself of Sex, also: because it will only be that much Better after your Fast is over: because all Parts of the Body Work Better.

15-02 [_] Moreover, concerning a Male Body, if you Endure until your whole Body is Cleaned Out of all Waste Matter, you will easily be Able to Maintain an Erection for Hours at a Time, as if you were Younger than a Teenager. Therefore, all Impotent Men should Especially be Interested in Fasting, which is a Guaranteed Cure if all Organs are in Place.

15-03 [_] Furthermore, if you Suffer with some Sexual Disease, Fasting is the Surest Cure, and it is Drug-free, Doctor-free, Hospital-free, and Tax-free. Indeed, there is Strong Evidence that Proper Fasting will also Cure AIDS, which is perhaps the Worst of Sexual Diseases. Therefore, if you have HIV-AIDS, be Sure to Follow the RULES for FASTING Closely: because your Immune System is already run down. †‡

15-04 [_] Moreover, I Recommend a Raw Food Diet, only, after Fasting: because that will Assist your Immune System, and especially if you get some Exercise and do a lot of Praying. In other Words, Try to Live on nothing but Raw Sweet Fruits, Raw Green Leaves, and a few Raw Nuts — all of which have been Grown by **"The LUSCIOUS All-Mineral Organic Method of Gardening,"** even as it is within ALL of those **"GLORIOUS Swanky Hotels Castles and Fortresses!" (Beautiful Planned City States for WISE Intelligent Well-Educated People with Common Sense and Good Understanding!)** Indeed, if you do not have one near to you, you should do your Best to SELL my Inspired Books, whereby you can Work Up some Interest in it. Otherwise, you will have to go on Suffering without the 5,000+ Good Reasons and Great Advantages for Building all such Swanky Fortresses. {See: **"The Right Design for Living!" (A List of Great Advantages for Building Beautiful Planned City States!) By The Worldwide People's Revolution!®** Book 012.}

15-05 [_] Remember that those MediSINZ are very Expensive, and Totally Unnecessary, if you Follow the Proper RULES for FASTING! Also, Remember that a Moderate Amount of Physical Exercise, early during the Cool Time of the Morning, in the Sunlight and Fresh Air, also Helps to Build Up your Immune System, as well as Positive Thinking about the Good Reasons and Great Advantages for Building those Beautiful Planned City States, which have Zero Great Disadvantages. Be Cheerful. After all, your Life is at Stake. Therefore, Stop Picking on other People, and Live in Peace. Be Thankful for all Good Things. Help other People. Pray to God. Study my Inspired Books. Share them with Friends. Make more Friends by doing Good for them.

— Chapter 16 —

HOW to take an ENEMA while Fasting

16-01 [_] First of all, you need to Understand what an Enema IS, which is an Internal Flushing or Rinsing of the Lower Bowels with Pure Spring Water through the Hole of the Anus, by Means of LOW Water Pressure through a Soft Tube, Hose, Pipe, Gourd, or Special Container with a Glass Funnel that is gently Inserted into the Anus, as a Person lies down on his or her Back, with his or her Buttocks lifted up by Means of Pillows, or by extending the Feet over the Head while resting on his or her Shoulders in Bed.

16-02 [_] In other Words, "BUTTS UP," as they say in the Military, for a "Bicycle Pedaling Exercise in the Air with your Feet," except that your Feet should be up and over your Head: so that your Buttocks are Spread Apart, and your Anus is fully Exposed, which also needs to be Thoroughly Oiled with Olive Oil or Mineral Oil before you Attempt to GENTLY Insert that Well-oiled Tube, Soft Hose, Soft Rubber Pipe, Prepared Gourd, or Smooth Glass Funnel, after RELAXING the Anus Muscles, which just Naturally Contract when Touched; but, Patience will Prevail, and Especially if this is done in Private, which is the Preferred Plan.

16-03 [_] However, if you are Old and Unable to Help yourself, you should Ask for Help, in spite of the Humiliation of it all: beCause it is far less Humiliating than being Examined and Inspected and Probed by Doctors and Nursexes in Horsepiddles, who may be more Interested in your Sex Organs, than in your Good Health. (I personally had one Medical Doctor play with my Sex Organs for about 20 Minutes when I was just a Teenager, who called it a "Physical Exam.") Moreover, that Tube or Funnel must have a SHUT-OFF Valve: so that you can STOP the Water from Running whenever you Want to, which will most likely be whenever you Feel too much Pressure within your Bowels. Otherwise, you would have to have someone else Assist you to take such an Enema, and they would simply pour a *little* Lukewarm Water into the Funnel at a Time from a Pitcher, even as they did in the City of Nineveh, some 2,400 Years Ago.

16-04 [_] However, since an Enema is such a PRIVATE and Personal Affair, it is less Em-BARE-assing (Embarrassing) to have a Proper Setup for taking an Enema, which is to use a Soft Rubber Tube with a Shut-off Valve near to the End of it. Indeed, without some Assistance, you will almost need a Special Waterproof Bed, plus at least a Secure Hook in the Ceiling of your House, or on the Wall beside your Bed, with a Rope attached to the Hook at one End, and the Enema Bottle, Bucket, Bag or Funnel attached to the other End, which allows it to Hang from the Ceiling to within one foot above your Anus: so that the Water Pressure is Minimized in the Hose or Tube that runs into your Anus, which is commonly called your Asshole, or Butt Hole.

16-05 [_] Yes, you also need to Understand that the Inside of your Bowels are very Tender, and that you can Injure them by Washing Out the Delicate Lining of the Rectum; and therefore, Cause an Infection or Eruption through the Rectum, which could Prove to be rather Deadly. Therefore, you do not Want to use a Conventional Tube that is used on a Standard Hot Water Bottle, nor Enema Bottle: because the Tube is far too Small, and therefore the Water Pressure is far too Great, and especially if the Water Bottle is held up much higher than your Body, which Increases the Water Pressure in the Tube, which is how it is done in most Hospitals, or Horse Piddles, where Medical Doctors have about as much Common Sense and Good Understanding as a Farmer's Cow might have: because they do not even See what is Happening!

16-06 [_] However, after taking dozens of Enemas, I Learned the DIFFICULT WAY how to do it Riit: beCause I managed to Wash OUT some of the Lining of my Bowels, which Required another 2 Weeks of Fasting for it to Heal up; and I was using a Standard American-made Enema Bottle, and was following Standard Medical Procedures at that Time, even as they are presently doing in all American Hospitals, as far as I know.

16-07 [_] Therefore, when it comes to giving Enemas, the Modern Medical Establishment is still in the "Dark Ages," you might say: because of not OBSERVING what comes Out of the Bowels of People to whom they are Administering Enemas. However, if you See any White Raw Flesh, or Mucus Membrane from your Intestines in your Stool, or in your Portable Potty (which can be nothing more Expensive than a Used 5-gallon Pickle Bucket with a Toilet Seat on Top of it), you must Understand that you are doing WRONG: because no such Mucus Membrane should be there, ever!

16-08 [_] Indeed, you must AIM that Tube or Funnel into your Anus at the same ANGLE as your Rectum, being PARALLEL with the Rectum, as if your Fingers were slipping into a Glove, or as if you were slipping one Oiled Finger into your Anus, in Order to Discover the Correct Angle while in the Exact same Position as you will be while Administering the Enema to yourself; or, while anyone else is doing it, who must have this same Understanding of what is Happening, which is much less Dangerous if one Assistant is using a Biblical GOURD with a Well-oiled Hole at the small End of it, whereby that Part of the Gourd can be Inserted into the Anus an Inch or 2 at the most, just passed the Sphincter Muscle at the Opening of the Anus, whereby Water can be Gently Poured into the Rectum. {NOTE: You might have to Oil up your Finger with a Rubber Glove on, and Work your Finger into the Anus, just to get it to Relax enough to Open Up and allow the Small End of the Oiled Gourd or Smooth Funnel into it. The Sphincter Muscle will Relax enough to Allow the Tube or whatever to pass through the Hole, if you give it Time to do so. (Remember that some Perverted Men actually Insert their Engorged Penises into the Anuses of other Men, which is called Sodomy, which is a Forbidden Sexual Act by God, who Allowed and Authorized Natural Ancient Greek Sex between Men, which is now called "Frot Sex," which you can read about in www.Man2ManAlliance.org for the Proof.) Therefore, if the Anus can Tolerate that Kind of Abuse, it can easily Tolerate a one-half-inch Tube, or even a 3/4th-inch Gourd. I much Prefer the Smooth Glass Funnel with a half-inch Opening, which is easy to Clean with Hot Water and Dish Soap, and Inspect it afterwards. However, it does Require both Hands to Operate it: because one Hand must be used to slowly pour out a Pint or more of Warm Water into the Funnel as it runs into the Rectum.}

16-09 [_] Meanwhile, if you do stick your Finger into your Rectum, make Sure that your Fingernail is Trimmed Back: so as to not make a Hole in your Rubber Glove, nor Scratch your Rectum; and, that you also Feel around Inside of your Rectum for any Lumps that might be Attached to the Inside of the Lining of your Rectum; and Notice that all such Lumps will Loosen Up and Detach themselves as you continue to Fast: because it is a Part of the Elimination Process of the Human Body, which is Able and Willing to Eliminate all Lumps from Head to Toe, if you just give to your Body a CHANCE to do its Homework, or House Cleaning. Moreover, you should not Attempt to Rip any Lumps Out with your Finger: because you might Damage the Lining of your Rectum. Just be Patient, and let Nature do its Thing as it will, while you Assist it with Patience.

16-10 [_] Indeed, you can REJOICE over the Fact that you will not Need any Colonectomy, Hysterectomy, Mastectomy, Breastectomy, Appendectomy, nor whatever other –ectomy: because all Lumps will simply DISAPPEAR! However, whenever you are Eating, or even Drinking Juices, Beer, Wine, or Eating any Kind of Foods, the Body will not make any Effort to get Rid of such Lumps: because the Body does not get the Message that you are Fasting, unless you are Actually Fasting, even as Moses was Fasting. {See *Deuteronomy 9:9 and 18,* and Understand that your Body is much Smarter than you are: because it Strictly Follows Natural LAWS, which you are most likely completely Ignorant of: because such Laws are not Taught to anyone in **"The Public School of IGNERUNT FQLZ!" (HOW we have been GRAATLEE DISEEVD!)**, Book 024. Therefore, just Trust your *Bible* to be Correct concerning those Points of Doctrines, and you will be a whole lot Wiser. Indeed, it Requires 3 to 4 Days of Fasting on NOTHING BUT AIR, just for the Body to get the Message that you are Truly and Sincerely FASTING, at which Time the Body will Determine for itself which Organ needs its Assistance, FIRST, and then it will go to Work to Remove any Unwanted Obstructions; and, at Last, after the Body has all Internal Organs in Perfect Condition, the Body will go to Work on less Vital Organs, such as the Skin, with the Skin of your Face being the LAST Part to Heal up Perfectly: beCause it is something that you can See in the Mirror of Truths, in Order to Judge whether or not you Need to Continue Fasting, take a Flush with Fruit Juices, or just take an Enema, which alone will Dramatically Change the Looks on your Face, if your Bowels are Relieved of X-amount of Accumulated Poisons, which Poisons can be so Poisonous that you will be as Weak as a Chicken, until those Poisons are Removed by Water; and once they are Thoroughly Removed, you will think that you might be Related with Samson, himself, who was Perhaps the Strongest Man who ever Lived, who Adhered to a very STRICT Nazirite DIET. See *Numbers 6.*}

16-11 [_] Therefore, when such Amazing Strength comes into your Body, as if it came from the Air that you Breathe, you should Rejoice in the Goodness of God, and give to him all of your Praise: because it was nothing that you did that made you Strong, nor Healthy, nor Happy — except to simply Cooperate with the Laws of Nature, which is your Duty. Indeed, you only STOPPED INTERFERING with the Work of your Creator, and you only Denied yourself of your Lusts, which Required Willpower that God gave to you: beCause of his Grace and Mercy, for which you should also Thank him, alone: because no one can give to himself that Grace, which Explains WHY that so many People FAIL with their Fasting: beCause they do not give to GOD all of the Credit and Glory for his Goodness, and how he Created every Body in such a Way that it can Heal itself, when left alone to do its Good Work; or, when Assisted to do its Good Work, by Eating God's Sweet Juicy Fruits, none of which were made by People.

16-12 [_] Indeed, People are so Vain that they want to take Credit to themselves for their own Healing, the same as many Athletes Try to take the Glory for their Successes in Winning Races or whatever Sports that they are engaged in, not Realizing that without the Assistance of God, such Acts would have never been Possible; and, without Good Health, which comes from Cooperation with God's Laws, they could not Win any Race, nor any other Game.

16-13 [_] In Fact, if such a Person is going to Praise anyone other than God, he or she should be Praising his or her Parents: because, without Healthy Bodies, Parents cannot Produce Healthy Children: because every Tree Produces Seeds According to its Health, and so do People. Therefore, Knowing that Fact of Life, we can Understand that there will never be a Winning Athlete Produced by Sickly, Degenerated Parents; nor has there ever been such a Winning Athlete: because it would be Impossible. {See the Stories of Adam, Enoch, Noah, Abraham, Isaac, Jacob, Joseph, Moses, Joshua, Samson, David, Jonathan, Solomon, and many other Biblical Characters for the Proof. In Fact, Moses Reminded us of those Facts, when he wrote: *"All of the Commandments, which I Command you this Day, shall you Observe to Do: so that you might Live, and Multiply, and go in and Possess the Land that the Creator Swore to your Fathers. And you shall Remember all of the Journey and the Lessons that you Learned while the Creator your Supreme Ruler Led you for these 40 Years in the Wilderness, in Order to Humble you, to Prove you, to Test your Spirits, and to Learn what was in your Hearts, whether or not you would Love and Obey his Commandments. And thus he Humbled you, and Allowed you to Hunger, which is like Fasting; but, the Effect is much Slower; and he Fed you with Manna, which you did not know about, neither did your Fathers know about it, nor even Hear about it: so that he might make you to Know that Man does not Live by Foods, alone; but, by every Word that proceeds out of the Mouth of the Creator God does Man Live. Moreover, your Clothing did not wax Old on you, neither did your Feet Swell for a Lack of Nourishment, nor for Excessive Nourishment, even for those 40 Years. Furthermore, you shall also Consider it in your Hearts, that, as a Man Chastens his Son, and Corrects him with a Switch, even so the Creator your Supreme Ruler Chastens you According to his own Wisdom, in his own Way, in his own Time, and in his own Chosen Place, in Order to bring you to Perfection for either Good or Evil. Therefore, you shall Learn to Love and Obey the Commandments of the Creator your Supreme Ruler, in Order to Walk in his Ways, and to Fear him, and to Obey him: because the Creator your Supreme Ruler will bring you into a Good Land, even into a Land of Brooks of Running Water, of Fountains and Springs of Water that gush out of the Hills and run through Valleys — a Land of Wheat, Barley, Oats, Corn and Rye — a Land of Grapevines, Fig Trees, Pomegranates, Dates, Apples, Peaches, Pears, Apricots, Plums, Cherries, and Berries, as well as all Kinds of Citrus Fruits, which are Good for Cleansing your Bowels — a Land of Olives, Olive Oil, Nut Trees, and Honey in Abundance; a Land wherein you shall Eat Food without Scarceness: because you shall not Lack anything; a Land whose Stones are like Iron, and out of whose Hills you may Dig Copper and Tin for making Brass, and Iron for making Steel, you might say, a Land with an Abundance of Natural Resources, both above and below the Ground. Therefore, when you have Eaten until you are Full, then you shall Remember to Bless and Thank the Creator your Supreme Ruler for all of the Goodness of that Blest Land, which he alone has Given to you: because you could have been Born in any other Land, among any other People, even in some Cursed Land in Africa or Asia, where they have not Learned about the Laws of their Creator. Therefore, be Aware that you do not Forget the Creator your Supreme Ruler, nor Mock him by not Obeying his Commandments, his Judgments, his Statutes, his Ordinances, and his Rules, which I Command to you this Day — lest when you have Eaten, and are Full of Foods, and have Built Goodly Houses for yourselves, and Live therein; and when your Herds and Flocks Multiply, and your Silver and Gold are Multiplied, and all that you have has Multiplied; and then your Hearts are lifted up with Great Pride, and you Forget the Creator your Supreme Ruler, who brought you forth, Out of the Land of Egypt, from the Household of Bondage and Tax Slavery; who Led you through that Great and Terrible Wilderness, wherein were Fires,*

Poisonous Serpents, Scorpions, and Drought, where there was no Water; who brought forth Water for you out of a Rock of Flint; who Fed you in the Wilderness with Manna, which your Fathers did not know anything about: so that he might Humble you by Reducing your Lusts and Limiting your Foods, so that he might Prove you and Test you, in Order to do you Good at your Latter End, at the End of the Ages, when he will make some of you Rulers with him within his Holy Kingdom, which will be Established over all of the Nations of the Earth. Therefore, let each of you Remember those Things, lest you say in your Heart: 'My power and the might of my own hands have gotten this wealth for me.' But, you shall Remember the Creator your Supreme Ruler: because it is he who has Given to you Power, in Order to get Wealth, and all that you have: so that he might Establish his Covenant with you, which he Swore to your Fathers that he would Give it to you, as it is this Day. And it shall be, that if you at all do Forget the Creator your Supreme Ruler, who has Blest you, and Walk after other Rulers, and Serve them, and Pay Taxes to them, and even Worship them — I Testify against you this Day that you shall Surely Perish as a Nation, even as the Nations that the Creator has Destroyed from in front of your Face, so shall you also Perish: beCause you would not be Obedient to the Voice of the Great Creator, your Supreme Ruler." — NMV of Deuteronomy 8.}

16-14 [_] Now, as you can Perceive, giving to yourself an Enema is a rather Frustrating Procedure, even if you have the Right Equipment, in Order to do it Correctly: because it is Difficult (if not Impossible for certain People) to hold up the Water Bottle, Funnel, or whatever, while at the same Time you Control the Water and let it into your Rectum. In other Words, it Requires Practice; and even then you are likely to SPILL some Water, or even let Water and Waste Matter out of your Bowels, before you can manage to get yourself on a Bucket or Toilet. {NOTE: I Recommend using a Bucket of some Kind, in Order to make it Possible for you to Scientifically Examine whatever has come out of you, both to See it and to Smell of it: beCause it was that Deathly Morbid Filth that was Tormenting you so much — NOT my Inspired Words of Provable Truths — which Filth is now still Tormenting you, IN AS MUCH AS any of it is still Lodged within you. Therefore, in Order to Remove any Doubts about what Kind of FILTH that it was that was Tormenting you, you must See it and Smell of it; but, do not Taste of it, nor Eat it, lest you should DIE from it, even if you are Starving to Death: beCause there are any Number of Wild Green Leaves that can be Eaten, or at least Wild Nuts, Roots, or something that only an Aborigine of Australia would know much about, if he were left alone in the Woods for a few Years. Nevertheless, you can now Prepare for such a Famine, by Stocking Up on Canned Groceries, Dried Fruits, Vacuum-packed Frozen Nuts, Vacuum-packed Whole Grains (which you can Sprout, if you have an Excessive Amount of Fresh Water to "Waste," which can be put around Edible Plants), and all Kinds of Hermetically-sealed Garden Seeds. However, you must Remember that WATER will be the Primary Substance for Survival, and IT will be so Scarce during a Great Famine, that you will Gnash your Teeth with Great REGRET, if you do not Build a LARGE Swanky Cistern or 2 for Water Storage: because it Requires at least 10 gallons of Water per Day, just to Grow Enough Food to Survive, even if you are only Sprouting it: because Sprouts have to be Rinsed Off 3 to 4 Times per Day, and especially if the Weather is Hot. However, Sprouted Wheat, for Example, can be used to make a very Delicious Bread, which is Baked by Solar Power, or Baked very slowly in a Dutch Oven. In other Words, NOW is the Time to Practice such Arts for Survival, NOT after the Famine comes: because you need to Learn HOW to Survive on those Wild Edibles, just to Learn that almost any "Domesticated" Food is Superior to any Food in the Wild; and just one 5-gallon Bucket of Good Honey could see you through a very LONG Famine, if you just Nibbled on it, each Day. But, Fresh WATER or Fruit Juice is the most Important Substance to Concentrate your Attention on: because, after Air, you cannot Live without Water, if only to Wash Out that Dung Bucket, once per Day, if you do not have a Place to Squat under a Tree: because of Living in some Filthy Stinking City of Massive Confusion, where you might be Fined for such an Act, or even Imprisoned. For Example, in Singapore, you could be Sentenced to 4 Years of Hard Labor, after being Lashed with a Whip, until you Wet your Panties, just for Urinating somewhere along the Street. Therefore, the Wise Person will THINK about what he or she would Do if the Worst Case should come on him or her.}

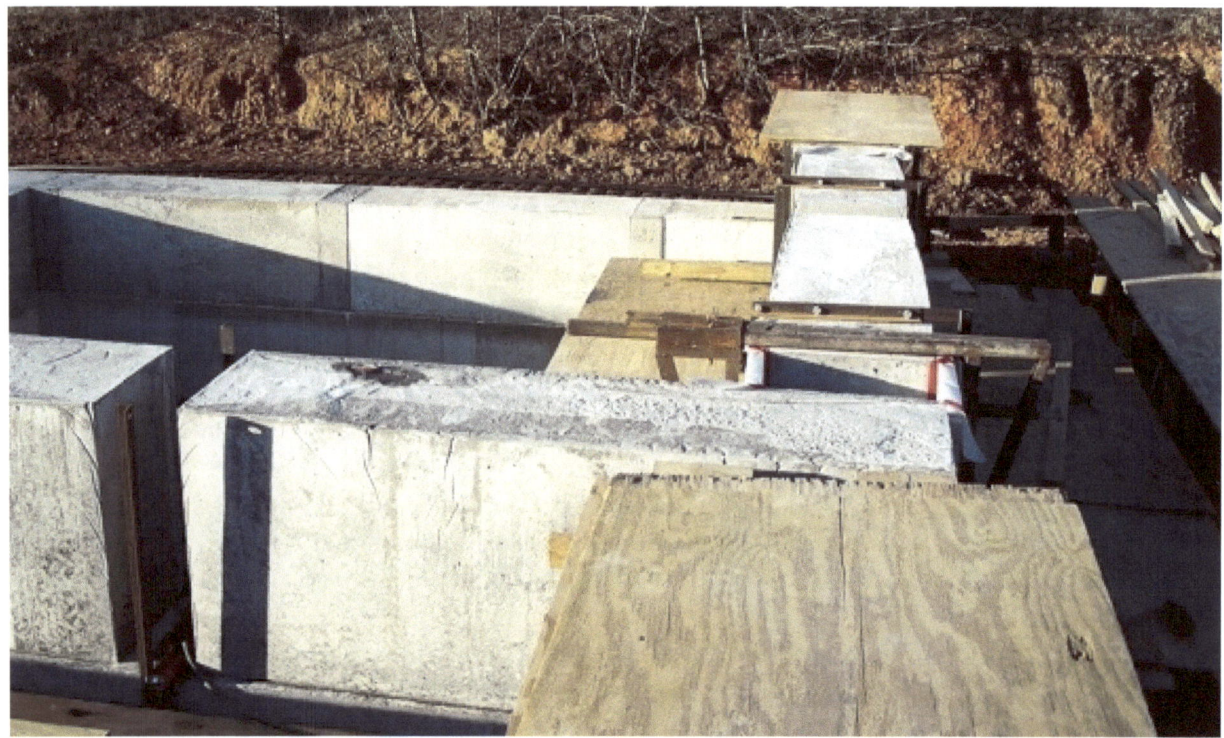

{NOTE: This Photo shows most of the Seventh Tier of our 100,000-gallon Cistern, which was built with large and small Concrete Blocks, in 8 Tiers, which have lapping Joints. It required 7 Years of Hard Work, which you can Learn all about in: **"The LUSCIOUS All-Mineral Organic Method of Gardening!"** — which contains many Photos with Explanations. I personally did most of the Work by myself on the last 4 Tiers. You can see one of the Small Concrete Forms set up at the far end of the 60-feet-long Ramp, which I used to Wheel over the Concrete in an Army Wheelbarrow, which we also used to Move more than 66,666,666 Pounds to Build our 98% Rock Houses, including our Retirement Home, in Mexico, which has about 6,000 square feet of Floor Space, for which you can find many Photos with Explanations in: **"What is WRong with those Professing Christians?" (A Self-Examination of the Heart of the Body of Good Government!) By The Worldwide People's Revolution!® Book 002.**}

16-15 [_] Now, after you let X-amount of Water from the Enema Bottle into your Rectum, your Body will Naturally Want to Reject it, or Expel it, and Especially if you Stand Up. {NOTE: You may Test the Temperature of the Enema Water by putting your Elbow into the Water, which should be Warm; but, neither Hot nor Cold, even though Cold is Better than too Hot.}

16-16 [ ] Therefore, your Waste Bucket needs to be beside of the Bed, so that you can get onto it as quickly as possible, before you "Explode." That is, before you Mess on your Bed, and Stink Up the Whole House! Moreover, you will also need to be in a Room that can be Aired Out: because it is almost certain to get very Odious, and especially if you have not done much Fasting, before now: because there is most likely several Pounds or Kilos of some very Ancient Morbid Matter that is Stored Up within your Bowels, which will Require a Month or more of Fasting, in order to Dislodge it and Move it Out by Force of Contractions of the Bowels. Yes, it has been in your Bowels for many Years, giving to you Bad Breath, Underarm Odors, Bad Dreams, Cramps, Aches, Headaches, Back Pains, Leg Aches, Colds, Flqz, Diarrheas, and who knows what else — all for a Lack of Fasting and a Natural Diet of Fruits, Clean Green Leaves, and a few Raw Nuts.

16-17 [ ] Nevertheless, most People will Postpone their Fasting, even though they now Know for a Fact what is Causing their Ailments: because they have so many Bills to Pay, and no Time for Fasting nor Praying. Indeed, we have a near Naaber, who is now Dying with Cancer; and yet he still Persists with his Eating and Smoking Habits: because, "if Medical Doctors do not know how to cure cancers, it is for sure that you do not know how," he says; and yet many other People have found that Fasting, when Combined with a Natural Diet, is their one and only Sure Cure, for which many Books have been Printed and Published — most of which are now Obsolete, or no longer in Print: because almost no one has any Faith in Fasting, nowadays; and even if they do, they do not have Time for it, they say; but, when a Person is Confined to a BED: because of his or her Cancer, you would think that he or she would Realize that he or she has nothing but Time for Fasting and Praying: because he or she is about to Meet with his or her Maker for Judgment and an Assignment to this Place or to that other Place, where he or she can Learn the Truth by Means of more Suffering.

16-18 [ ] Otherwise, for what Purpose would such Suffering Occur? Indeed, if it were not for Good Lessons, God could have given to each of us a Body that has NO Nerves, and therefore NO Pains, even if a Lion is Eating Holes in our Backsides. However, **PAINS are WARNING VOICES, Warning us about something that is WRONG.** For Example, if someone is Standing on your Foot, Causing you to have Pains, the Cure is to REMOVE that Person from Standing on your Foot — not to take a thousand Dollars-worth of Pain-killing Pills! Indeed, some Fools might Suggest that you should AMPUTATE your Foot, do Meditation Exercises, or Suck on your Thumb; but, the one and only Reasonable Solution is to REMOVE that Idiot who is Standing on your Foot, who should Know that it is WRong to do so. However, Strangely enough, there are X-amount of Medical Doctors who Suggest that if you have Pains, that you should simply KILL those Pains with Medications, with Opium, Heroin, or Morphine — rather than Discover whatever is CAUSING the Pains, which is usually Pressure on the Nerves: because of Internal FILTH, which Causes CONGESTION, or a BUILD UP of Slime within a certain Area of the Body.

16-19 [ ] In other Words, when we Fast, the entire Body SHRINKS, and thus much of the Internal Pressure is Relieved, no matter where it is; but, especially within the Bloodstream, which is Evident by the Appearance of the Blood Vessels that are seen on People's Hands, whose Blood Vessels EXPAND whenever they Eat or do some Exercising, while their Blood Vessels CONTRACT whenever they Stop Eating for a few Days, and also Stop Exercising.

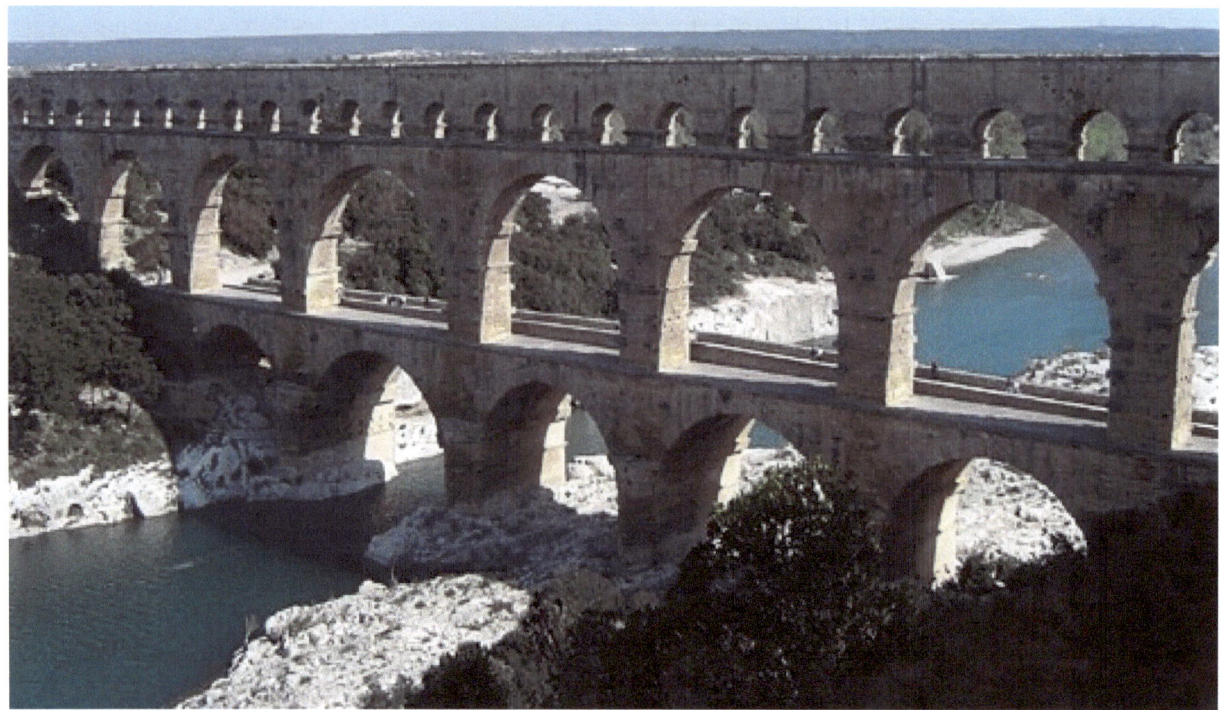

{NOTE: This is one of many Ancient Roman Aqueducts, which was Constructed without the Assistance of Rock-cutting Machines, Trains, nor Modern Cranes. Notice the True Stone Arches, which are very Strong. No Independent Jackass could have ever Accomplished such a Great Feat. See: **"The Loathsome Burdens of the Independent Jackasses!" (A New Approach for Solving our Massive Problems!)**, Book 051, plus: **"Seven Great Armies of Working Soldiers!" (HOW to Provide a Way for everyone to WORK: so as to Eliminate Poverty, Crimes, Drug Abuses, Prisons and Unnecessary Taxes!) By The Worldwide People's Revolution!®** Book 015.}

16-20 [_] Moreover, if you Fast Long Enough — as in 40 Days — your Blood Vessels will simply DISAPPEAR, like those of a little Baby! And your BIG Muscles will also Disappear, while your Strength will INCREASE by perhaps 10 Times! Therefore, Strength does not come from Eating, as most People Vainly Imagine; but, it comes from being Free from all Internal Obstructions: because a Person can be Incredibly Strong without Eating anything for 40 Days, as Moses Proved, who walked down from Mount Sinai after Fasting for 40 Days. Indeed, he obviously only Drank Water after his Fasting, which alone Gave to him his Strength: because it FLUSHED OUT his Bowels, and therefore FLUSHED OUT any Poisons, Excess Mucus, or whatever his Body decided to get Rid of: because the Body would not get Rid of any Precious Thing that might be Good for it, which it ought to Retain: because that would be Insane!

16-21 [_] Indeed, the Body Knows what is Best for itself, and it KEEPS whatever it Wants, while it Tries to get RID of whatever it does not Want, if you give to it a Chance to do its Thing, which is to Eliminate any Unwanted Garbage. Therefore, it is Ridiculous for Medical Doctors to take Urine Samples to be Tested for whatever might be in the Urine, when the Source of their Problems is found on their Dinner Plates!

16-22 [_] However, we all Know that 10 People can Eat the very same Kinds of Foods, and yet come up with Different Ailments: because of Genetic Inheritances, and Living Habits. Otherwise, everyone in the World might Suffer with the very same Ailments. However, no 2 People on this Earth can Eat just alike, even if they Want to: because the Elements of each Bite of Food will be Different, not to mention the Thoughts of the People who are Eating it, which might have a Greater Bearing on the Final Outcome: because Good Thoughts can Produce certain Beneficial Acids, while Evil Thoughts can Produce certain Detrimental Acids, and some Evil Thoughts can even KILL YOU!

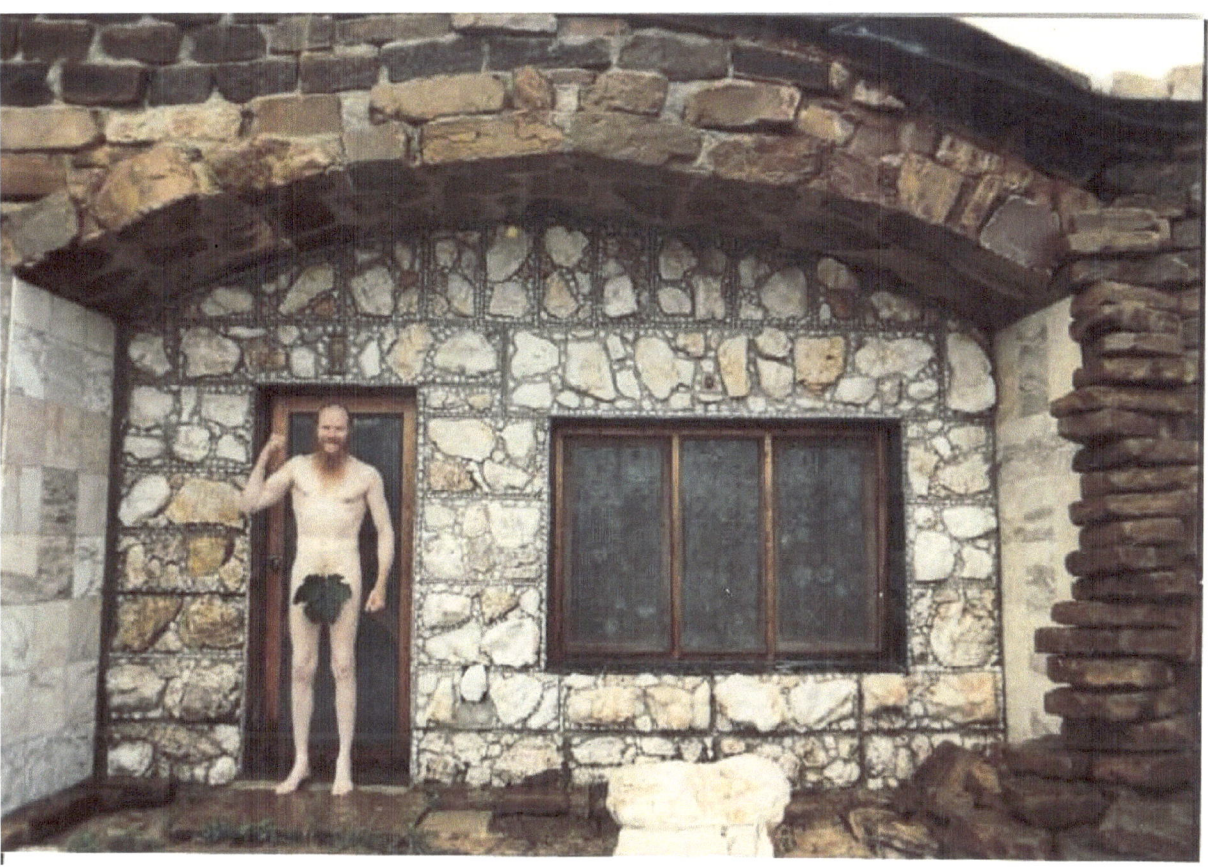

{FOOTNOTE: Those Slender Legs and Strong Knees have Won hundreds of Races. It required 3 Months of Moderate Work to Install the White Quartz Crystal Rocks on the Facing Walls of our 98% Rock Houses. Notice the one large Lintel Rock over the Brazilian Agate Windows, which is about 8 feet long. [You can see many Photos of those Agate Windows in Spectacular Natural Colors in: **"The New MAGNIFIED Version of ISAIAH in Plain English!" (The Understandable Version of the Book of Isaiah!)**, Book 044.] My Brother Vern and I put that 800+-pound Lintel Rock up there by Hand, without any Forklift, after Fasting for a Month or so. Notice the Onyx Vase above the Doorway, which is Permanently Set in another Lintel Stone, which we also set up there by Hand. Also notice the 20,000$ Quartz Crystal Stone in front of the Windows, on the Ground, which we Discovered for Free with a Pick and Shovel! Those Crystal Stones make Permanent Siding on the Houses. Tornadoes Shy Away from them, as well as the Hail-proof Roof, which has 400+ Tons of Rocks and Concrete to Strengthen it. Notice that after Fasting for 314 Days during 14 Months, I did not become an Invalid!}

16-23 [_] Indeed, it is a Common Thing for certain People to Hear Bad News, and then Suffer with a Heart Attack, Stroke, Seizure, Cramps, or whatever; but, just a short Prayer can keep that Person Alive! Moreover, an Enema can also Relieve the Pressure within the Bowels, and Prevent a Stroke, Heart Attack, Seizure, Cramp, or whatever, if it is Combined with Praying and Fasting. Therefore, whenever you get Upset — or just Lose your Appetite — that, my Friend, is the Time to FAST and PRAY: because you will only do Damage to yourself if you Eat: because your Body is Trying to tell you to FAST, just by taking away your Appetite!

16-24 [_] Therefore, do not Listen to some Ignorant Fool, who Suggests that you will get Weak if you do not Eat: because, *"To every Thing there is a Season, and a Time for every Purpose under Heaven; a Time to be Born, and a Time to Die; a Time to be Strong, and a Time to be Weak; a Time to Plant, and a Time to Harvest; a Time to Wound, and a Time to Heal; a Time to Break Down, and a Time to Build Up; a Time to be Proud, and a Time to be Humble; a Time to Weep, and a Time to Laugh; a Time to be Boastful, and a Time to be Self-deprecating; a Time to Mourn, and a Time to Dance; a Time to be Honest, and a Time to be Dishonest; a Time to be Wise, and a Time to be a Fool; a Time to Cast Away Stones, and a Time to Gather Stones Together; a Time to Embrace, and a Time to Refrain from Embracing; a Time to Eat, and a Time to Fast; and Time to Gain, and a Time to Lose; a Time to Receive, and a Time to Give; a Time to Keep, and a Time to Cast Away; a Time to Tear Apart, and a Time to Sew Together; a Time to Speak, and a Time to keep Silent; a Time to Walk In, and a Time to Walk Out; a Time to Love, and a Time to Hate; a Time to make War, and a Time to make Peace; a Time to Murder, and a Time to Rescue; a Time to Defend, and a Time to Offend; a Time to be Aggressive, and a Time to Retreat; a Time to Taste, and a Time to Refrain from Tasting; a time to Smell, and a Time to Refrain from Smelling; a Time to Look, and a Time to Refrain from Looking; a Time to Reach In, and a Time to Pull Out; a Time to Stand Up, and a Time to Sit Down; a Time to Drill a Hole, and a Time to Plug a Hole; a Time to have Sex, and a Time to Refrain from having Sex; a Time to Report a Matter, and a Time to Cover it up; a Time to Dig in the Garden, and a Time to let the Soil Rest; a Time to Teach, and a Time to Learn; a Time to Add Spices, and a Time to Leave them Out; a Time to Cook, and a Time not to Cook; a Time to Clean House, and a Time to not Clean House; a Time to go to Town, and a Time to Stay at Home; a Time to Spend Money, and a Time to Save Money; a Time to Assist the Poor People, and a Time to Refrain from Assisting the Poor People; a Time to Assist the Rich People, and a Time to Refrain from Assisting the Rich People; a Time to Bury Treasures, and a Time to Dig Up Treasures; a Time to Reveal the Truth, and a Time to Hide the Truth; a Time to go to Court to Correct a Matter, and a Time to Refrain from going to Court; a Time to Judge, and a Time to not Judge; a Time to Condemn, and a Time to not Condemn; a Time to Sacrifice, and a Time to not Sacrifice; a Time to Share, and a Time to be Selfish; a Time to Remember, and a Time to Forget; a Time to Procrastinate, and a Time to not put it Off any longer; a Time to Make a Fire, and a Time to put Out the Fire; a Time to Bear a Burden, and a Time to Rest; a Time to Sleep, and a Time to get Up; a Time to Enjoy Pleasures, and a Time to Deny yourself of all Pleasures; a Time to Rejoice, and a Time to Grieve; a Time to go to Work, and a Time to Repose; a Time to Borrow, and a Time to Pay Back that which you have Borrowed; a Time to Loan, and a Time to Refrain from Loaning; a Time to Count the Cost, and a Time to not bother to Count the Cost; a Time to Forgive, and a Time to Hold a Grudge; a Time to get Revenge, and a Time to let God get Revenge for you; a Time to Bow Down, and a Time to Rise Up and take Over; a Time to be a Servant, and a Time to be a Master; a Time to Submit, and a Time to Command; a Time to Rule, and a Time to be Ruled; a Time to Breathe, and a Time to not Breathe; a Time to be Free, and a Time to be Captive; a Time to Preach the Truth, and a Time to Practice the Truths that your have been Preaching; a Time to Smile, and a Time to Frown; a Time to be Cheerful, and a Time to be Sober and Grave; a Time to Slow Down, and a Time to Speed Up; a Time to Freeze, and a Time to Heat; a Time to Steal, and a Time to Restore; a Time to Lie, and a Time to Tell the Truth; but, all of those Times are Subject to Circumstances, Conditions, and Situations — all of which are Determined by the Creator, who is Testing our Spirits, in Order to Discover which ones among us are Worthy to Govern this World with him within his Holy Kingdom: because there is a Time for Good and Evil Rewards, and only the Righteous People will be Blest with the Good Rewards: because they Chose to Do what is Right for themselves and others, According to the Laws and Rules of the Supreme Ruler. Therefore, Obey his Voice, and put the First Degree Murderers to Death: so that God might Judge them, and Assign them to Appropriate Places for them, where they can Learn their Lessons. Otherwise, they might be Assigned to Rule Over you after that Great Day of Profound Judgment, when every Knee will Bow, and every Tongue will Confess that there is a Time to Kill, in Order for God to get his Justice; but, only if you Know for a Fact that the Person has been Proven to be Guilty of First Degree Murder, and Confesses it, himself."* (See *The NMV of Ecclesiastes 3.*)

16-25 [_] Therefore, there is also a Time to take an Enema, which is just before you Decide to EAT; but, only IF you can Endure your Fasting for at least another 4 Days before you Flush Out your Bowels by Eating Fruits, or by Drinking Fruit Juices. Therefore, you are Faced with a very Perplexing Decision to make: because, if you do take an Enema, and then you cannot continue to Fast for another 3 or 4 Days, you will not have Successful Bowel Movements, such as you ought to have, and such as you should have if you Follow the RULES.

16-26 [_] Indeed, if you have Allowed certain Lusts for Foods into your Mind, and if you Feel very Tormented by the Filth that is Lodged within you, you will have a Great Desire to EAT; BUT, an Enema can Remove that Desire, by Relieving you of X-amount of Filth and Poisons, which would otherwise "Drive you Crazy," as they say.

16-27 [_] Moreover, it will be Difficult to Abstain from Enemas, once you Discover how Effective they are for Relieving you of those Torments that are Caused by Ancient Acids and Internal Filth. Indeed, many People continue to take Enemas for the Remainder of their Lives, which is also a very BAD Habit: because it is not Natural, Normal, nor Necessary.

16-28 [_] Likewise, other People get into the Bad Habit of using Chemical Laxatives, or even Natural Laxatives, to which they become Addicted, and cannot even have a Normal Bowel Movement without those Laxatives. Therefore, it is Advisable to only use Enemas and Laxatives when they are Absolutely Necessary, which is during your Fasting and Flushing Program; but, only IF you do it Correctly.

16-29 [_] Therefore, if you cannot give an Enema to yourself, you will have to call for Help from someone other than myself: because I do not particularly like such a Job, and would rather Shovel 10 Tons of Sand: because of the AWFUL SMELL of that Morbid Matter that will no Doubt come Out of your Bowels, if you have not done much Fasting, and are of an Age of 20

Years or more. Therefore, ask your Medical Doctor for some Help to take an Enema, whereby he might Discover the Truth of it.

16-30 [_] Now, I Hear someone, who is like an Innocent Lamb, bleat: "O Peacock, is it Right for Children to Fast for 30 to 40 Days, since their Bodies are much smaller than those of Adults? Moreover, why should Children have to take Enemas?"

16-31 [_] Well, O Lamb, in most Cases, Children are much more Internally Cleaner than Adults; and therefore, they will not need Enemas. However, because of Eating Unnatural Foods, the Bowels of Children can become BLOCKED by Super Sticky Foods, which can Cause HIGH Fevers, which can also be Relieved or even Eliminated by the Wise Use of Enemas. In Fact, that was the only Remedy for thousands of Years, among Enlightened People, who Understood that the Bowels are a PIPE System, which must not be Blocked by any Concentration of Filth. Indeed, you must Understand that there would not have been any other Way that the People of Nineveh could have kept themselves Alive, except to take Enemas when they Needed them.

16-32 [_] Otherwise, many of them would have Suffocated to Death in their own Slime, even as most Americans would do, right now, if they did not Eat nor Drink anything for 40 Days and 40 Nights. Moreover, because Children are not so full of Filth, they can Fast with greater ease than most Adults; but, only after 3 or 4 Days, after they have taken at least one Flush with Fruit Juices, or with just plain Immature Coconut Water, only.

16-33 [_] **Remember that it is Important to not Eat any Solid Foods after Flushing with Juices, if you Intend to go on Fasting:** because those Solid Foods will only Torment you, and Cause the same Uncomfortable Feeling that you had during your first 3 to 4 Days of Fasting. Therefore, you must Resist the Temptation to Eat any Fruits, or any other Solid Foods, after you Flush: because Fasting is really EASY after taking a Flush with Fruit Juices, only. Indeed, you will easily be Able to Fast for 4 to 5 Days after a Flush, at which Time you can tell yourself that anyone can Fast for 2 more Days, making a Total of 6 to 7 Days, at which Time you can Flush Out your Bowels, once again; and keep Extending the Days of Fasting and Flushing, until at last you can go for 20 Days or more without even taking Enemas nor Flushes: because the Bulk of the Filth will be Removed from your Body, which makes Fasting easier and easier as you Fast more and more, which is WHY that certain Indians in India can easily Fast for 40 Days or more: because their Bodies are Cleaner, and thus their Minds are less Tormented.

16-34 [_] Now, I Hear someone, who is like a Cricket, chirp: "O Peacock, if Fasting were so Effective for making People HOLY, how come those Skinny Africans are not Holy People, who often Starve to Death, being nothing but Skin covering Bones, you might say?"

16-35 [_] Well, O Critic, if you just Eat a very Small Amount of Food, your Body never does get the Message that you are Fasting; but, it just Assumes that more Food is coming down the Tubes, and Especially if you Plan on Eating: because your Thoughts can Determine the Reactions within your Bowels. In Fact, if I just tell myself that I am going to Fast, my Bowels simply LOCK UP, and I do not have any more Bowel Movements for 3 to 4 Days: because my Body Knows that it must Store Up as much Food as Possible: because I am going to Starve it by Self-denial, which someone might say is BAD; but, Moses might say that it is GOOD.

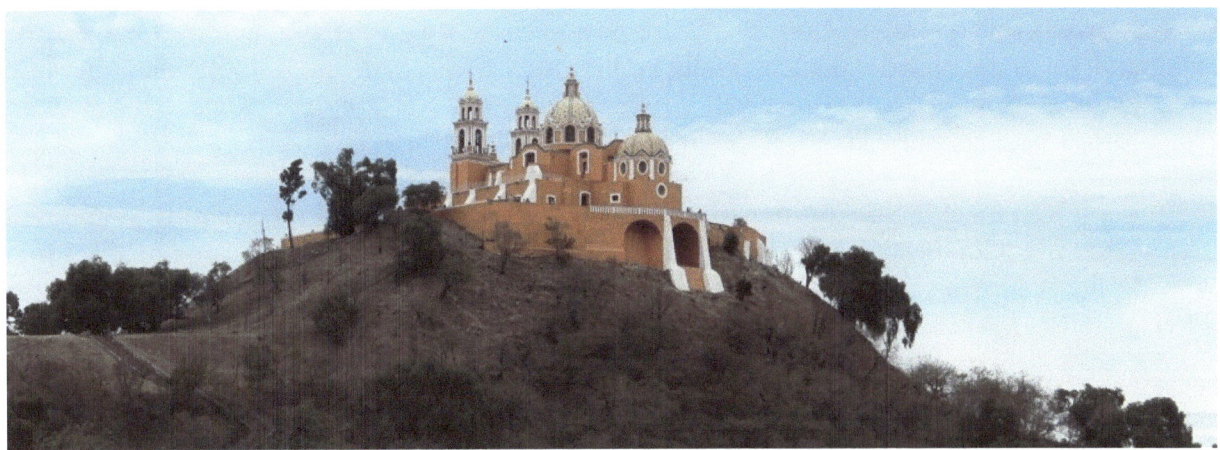

{FOOTNOTE: Zealots have built a Sanctuary on "Mount Sinai," whereby Moses can Fast more Comfortably the next Time around. Actually, no one Knows for Sure just WHERE Mount Sinai is Located, seeing that there is no Place to even Pitch a Tent over there in that Desert, much less Tents for 6 Million People: because most of the Ground is too Steep and Rocky. See Wikipedia.}

16-36 [_] However, just as soon as I go back to Eating, there is no Problem: because my Bowels begin to Work, once again. Therefore, during a Famine Situation, when there is very little if anything to Eat, you can also Expect your Bowels to LOCK UP and RETAIN whatever you have Eaten: because your Mind does have that much Effect on your Bowels. Therefore, that is all the more Reason WHY that everyone should have a GOOD Food Supply, such as a 7-Year Food Supply; but, Especially a GOOD Water Supply of no less than 25,000 Gallons per Person: because there are Friends and Relatives who will be BEGGING for some of your Water, just to take an Enema.

16-37 [ ] Now, I Hear someone, who is like a Buzzard, caw: "O Peacock, if Times get Bad, and there is little or no Fresh Water, is it OKAY to Use Swamp Water for taking an Enema?"

16-38 [_] Well, O Buzzard, you can Contract certain Diseases from Filthy Water, and you could even Kill yourself by taking such an Enema, if some Creature has Died in that Swamp; and therefore, it is not Wise to use it for any Purpose, until after you Filter it through Sand, and then BOIL it for at least 10 Minutes, after it gets to Boiling. Moreover, in Order to Filter it through Sand, you must Build a Proper Sand Box, which is about 3 feet high, wide, and long, or 3 feet Cubed; and put the Entrance Pipe for the Water in the Bottom of the Box, with the Outlet Pipe near the Top of the Box: because it is Necessary to Try to keep the Filth or Waste at the Bottom of the Box. Therefore, you must use a Clean 50-gallon Barrel, Tub, or Wooden Box that sits up on a Bench or Ramp, which is up above the Sand Box, which has a 2-inch Pipe coming out of the Bottom of the Barrel, with a Filter or Screen at the Head of the Pipe, just Inside of the Barrel, in Order to Try to Filter Out as much Heavy Material as possible, first; and then run that Pipe down to the Bottom of the Sand Box, and Seal it up with Caulking or the Correct Pipe Fittings; and then Patiently wait for the Water to Rise Up through the Clean Sand, which will Clean the Water as it Rises.

16-39 [_] However, if that Water does not Appear to be Clean, you must Filter it through another Sand Box, Remembering that Running Water is always more Pure than Stagnant Water in a

Swamp, or wherever. Nevertheless, in spite of how Clean it might Appear, do not Trust it to be Pure, until you have Boiled it; and then only Drink a very Small Amount of it for a Test: because it could have some Deadly Chemical Waste Products in it from the Anus of American Capitalism, which not only STINKS; but, it also Poisons everything around it.

16-40 [_] Therefore, if you do not See any Living Creatures in that Swamp Water, be Aware that it is Horribly Contaminated, and should not be Used for Drinking nor Cooking, even if you are Dying from Thirst. Remember that right NOW is the Time to get Set Up for Survival — NOT when the Rain STOPS!

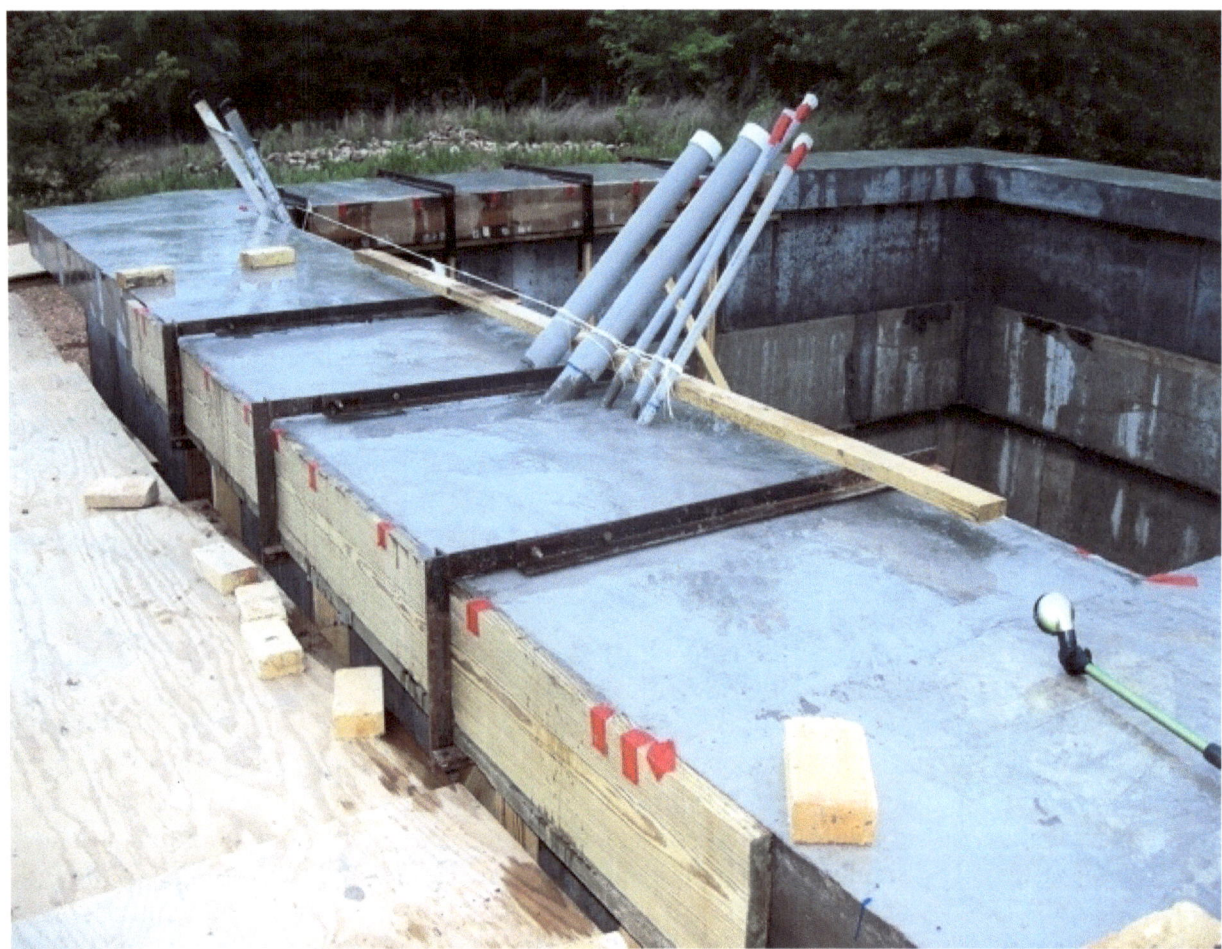

{FOOTNOTE: This Photo shows HOW I made the Concrete "Capstone" for the Walls of the 100,000-gallon Cistern, for making a Solid Concrete Pyramid Covering on Top of the Capstone. It took me 3 Days to Set Up the Forms, and Part of one Day to Mix and Pour the 2 Final Blocks, using a 130-feet-long Ramp. Trust me, it was lots of Fun, and Greatly Rewarding Work, until we got Underhandedly Robbed by Red Jew Bankers, who Judged the entire Project to be Valueless! Indeed, they Determined that it added NO Value whatsoever to the Property, which was also True for all of the other Permanent Buildings that we Constructed during 30 Years of Hard Labor, while Investing no less than 300,000$ in it! Yes, that is the Unjust Reward that we got for "Living in the greatest nation on the earth!" (Notice that "greatest nation" was not Capitalized, as in: "The Greatest Nation on the Earth": because it Falls far Short of that. However, let us Look at the Bright Side of this Issue, which I have already pointed out in: **"LIGHTNING Versus the Lightning Bug!" (HOW almost Everyone can become Moderately RICH, without Telling Any Lies nor Selling Any Trash!) By The Worldwide People's Revolution!®**, Book 001, which contains many Photos with Enlightening Explanations.}

16-41 [_] Also Remember that right NOW there are TRILLIONS of Gallons of Water just RUNNING AWAY into the Ocean of Forgetfulness: because almost no one is Concerned about any Great Famine that is Coming: because, "It has always Rained," they say. However, when that Great Famine does Come, it will take all of those Ignorant Fools by SURPRISE: because they have put their Trust in that Wicked, WICKED Anti-Christ False Cover-up Federal Government of Demon-possessed People in Low Places, who have only made Provisions for themselves, and NOTHING for the Masses of People, except for those almost Useless Dams and Reservoirs, which only have the APPEARANCE of an Abundant Water Supply.

16-42 [_] Indeed, if such Reservoirs are not Regularly Supplied with Rainwater, they Dry Up within ONE Year: because they are only Great Deceptions of the Mind, being WIDE and BROAD, like a Shallow Lake; but, usually not very Deep, being 20 to 50 feet Deep. Therefore, when a Huge City like Lost Angels, Californicate, uses ONE THIRD of a FOOT of that Water per Day, there is only a 150-Day Supply, unless it comes another Rain, or Snow Storm. Therefore, the Wise Person would get his or her own large Cisterns Prepared to hold the Rainwater that comes off of his or her Roof, if he or she Lives where it Rains very much — except that most Rainwater is Contaminated with Acids and Industrial Filth from the Smoke Stacks of Worldwide Capitalism, which is Blown by the Wind all over the Earth. In Fact, it was Reported just last Week that one of the most Contaminated Places on this Earth is found in the ARCTIC, where Polar Bears Try to Live!

16-43 [_] Therefore, if your Rainwater is not Crystal Clear; but, Appears like Piss Water, or Light Beer, be Aware that it is Full of Harmful Acids, which are no Good for Drinking, Cooking, nor even taking a Bath in: because the Skin Absorbs a Portion of whatever you put on it, including Mercury, Arsenic, Lead, Cadmium, and other By-products from Oil Refineries that Produce Gasoline for those Wonderful CARS that we all Love more than Life. †§

16-44 [_] Therefore, the next Time that you Turn the Key, in Order to Start the Car, just Remember that you are Contributing to Satan's Cause, which is to Destroy the Earth; and therefore, you are likely to be Destroyed with Satan and Sons, Incorporated, unless you REPENT, and Change your Lifestyle, and Help others to Build those **"GLORIOUS Swanky Hotels Castles and Fortresses,"** which have no Need for any such Vehicles: beCause they are Designed for LIVING! (See *Revelation 11, 17—18, and 22.*)

77

— Chapter 17 —

A Time for Weeping and Mourning!

17-01 [_] Some People would say that this should have been Chapter 01: because it is more Important than any Chapter within this Book: beCause True Repentance Begins with Feeling Sorry for Doing Wrong Things, and Especially for Directly Disobeying the Commandments of God — one of which is to Love our Naaberz as much as we Love ourselves, which we are not Doing when we Contaminate our Naaberz' Air, Water, and Land with Abominations like Gasoline, Motor Oil, and the Exhaust that comes Out of those Stinking Vehicles, including Airplanes, Ships, and Trains, even though the Least Harmful are those Trains: because they can Move a LOT of Tonnage with very little Energy — at least on Level Ground.

17-02 [_] Now, I Hear someone, who is like a Docile Cow, moo: "O Peacock, it is not Reasonable to Think that God put Natural Gases, Oils, Coals, and all such Good Things in the Earth, if he did not Want us to Use them."

17-03 [_] Trust me, many People will Check the above Box with an X: beCause of Believing that same Thing, including myself: beCause all such Good Things can be Used WISELY, if we have a Mind to do so. However, to Burn Up a Billion-year Supply of so-called "Fossil" Fuels within only 100 Years, is NOT Acting very Wisely: because the Great Great Grandchildren might need some Energy from all such Fuels, which would have been Saved for them, if we had Acted Wisely, and Built those **"GLORIOUS Swanky Hotels Castles and Fortresses!" (Beautiful Planned City States for WISE Intelligent Well-Educated People with Common Sense and Good Understanding!) By The Worldwide People's Revolution!®** Book 019. Indeed, those Cities are Self-air-conditioned, whereby they Automatically Heat and Cool themselves. Moreover, their Electricity is Generated by the WIND and Sunlight, or by Ox-power in an Emergency. Therefore, the Electric Elevators, Escalators, and Trains are not Polluting the Earth as much as a Dozen Cars per Fortress, even if it contains a Million People!

17-04 [_] O Elected King, if those Swanky Fortresses use Wind and Sunlight for Power, why Waste any Gas and Oil?

17-05 [_] Well, there are certain Heavy Machines — such as Bulldozers, Combines, Tractors, and Locomotives — that Burn Diesel Efficiently in Remote Places, where it is not Practical to use Electric-powered Machines, which is Especially True of Airplanes, most of which should be Grounded: because it is now Possible and most Practical for 99.99% of the People to Live within those Swanky Fortresses, while the other .01% can Live on the Water, if they Want to, seeing that it is their Tradition to do so: because they are Fishermen, Shipmasters, or whatever. Therefore, 99.99% of those Airplanes are not Needed, much less Wanted by Sane People: because they are the Worst of Polluters, which makes the United States Air Force the Chief Criminal in that DEPARTment. However, the Atlantic Ocean might have to Rise Up until Washington, District of Corruption, is Covered with Water, before we can get their Attention and Cooperation.

17-06 [_] O Elected King, I cannot Visualize any of those Politicians Weeping nor Mourning for the Sins of Americans, much less their own Sins: because they Judge themselves to be Superior to all other Nations. Therefore, it could be that they will have to be Cleaned Off of the Earth with Hydrogen Bombs, and Vladimir Putin is just the Man who could make that Happen with a Good Conscience: because he does not have much Respect for such Lying Hypocrites as one can Discover in the District of Criminals, in Washington. After all, they Profess to be "Christians," while Acting like Satan, himself.

17-07 [_] Well, with a Mentally Unstable Character like Donald Trumpeter in the Little White Outhouse, anything is Possible in the War Department of Death. After all, he is a Chief Bully, who is Repulsive to most Intelligent Educated People. Therefore, he could easily bring about a Situation that might call for Intercontinental Ballistic Missiles to be Dumped on 200 American Cities, just to Lower their PRIDE unto the Dust, which is Certainly a Just Cause for Weeping and Mourning for the Heavy Loss of many Innocent Ignorant People. Believe me, Judgment Day is Bound to Come, if we do not all REPENT, According to the LAW of Repentance, which Requires a Drastic Change of Mind and Heart and Living, without Seeking any Justifications for Wickedness, including the EVILS of Capitalism. {See www.Amazon.com for: **"The Nature of CAPITALISM!" (A List of the EVILS of CAPITALISM!) By The Worldwide People's Revolution!® Book 038.**}

17-08 [_] O Elected King, that is one Awful Sad Note to End a Book with, as if to say: REPENT or PERISH! Yes, it is an Ultimatum that I do not Like. However, when God gets Pissed Off with us for our Selfishness and Greed, we are in BIG Trouble! Indeed, Moses made it Clear in *Deuteronomy 8.* (See Chapter 16-13.) Therefore, it Sounds like we Americans are DOOMED!

17-09 [_] Well, as long as there is FAITH, HOPE, and LOVE, there is a Chance that the Majority of the People will Repent, and thus Decide to go to Work on the Construction of those **"GLORIOUS Swanky Hotels Castles and Fortresses,"** whereby we can be Saved from our MADNESS. After all, it is just a Matter of TIME when that Oil and Gas will RUN OUT, and then the Great Grandchildren will be Faced with the Exact same Problems to Solve — except that there will be NO Cheap Energy to Use for the Construction of any such Cities: beCause it will be in the Atmosphere, having been BURNED UP by Ignorant Selfish GREEDY FOOLS!

17-10 [_] O Elected King, I Sense that you are Correct — that we are our own Worst Enemies. Indeed, Vladimir Putin will not have to Dump any Bombs on us: because we will simply Destroy ourselves with our own Abominations. Perhaps the Chinese People will Weep and Mourn for us; but, I Doubt it. Who would have ever Thought that most Americans would Willingly Choose to Live in their Wooden / Plastic Firetrap Mouse-infested Cockroach Dens, as Opposed to Choosing to Live in **"Beautiful Swanky PALACES!"**?

— Chapter 18 —

The Conclusion

18-01 [_] Now, as you can See, not even this Book could Contain all of the Answers to all of your Questions about Fasting; and therefore, like it or not, I must make up another Volume, and perhaps even another one after that: because there are a LOT of Questions, even though many of those Questions are already Answered within other Books that I have written — such as: **"The Gospel According to our Elected King!" (The Good News from the Most Modern Perspective!)**, Book 013, plus: **"The New MAGNIFIED Version of the GOOD NEWS According to Saint JOHN!" (The Gospel According to Saint John Zebedee Boanerges in Plain English!)**, Book 062, and in: **"HOW to Become a HOLY Man!" (40 Good Reasons WHY People Should FAST and PRAY!) By The Worldwide People's Revolution!® Book 045.**

18-02 [_] Indeed, after reading about those Acid Rains, which Blow in the Wind all around the World, you might be Thinking that there is NO *Ideal* Place to Live; but, my Inspired Books are full of Surprises, even as this Book is full of Surprises for most People, who have never "red" any other Book about Fasting. Therefore, you must Exercise FAITH, Hope, Trust, Love, Patience, Persistence, Tolerance, Forgiveness, Longsuffering, and, most of all, COMMON SENSE; or else you will do your Fasting in such a Way that it will Discourage you from doing more of it, and then the Devil and your Naaberz will be LAUGHING at you, as if they could do it Better than you.

18-03 [_] However, the very Reason that they Laugh, is beCause they have never Done it; but, do not be Discouraged by that: because, when that Great Famine comes, Worldwide, they will be FORCED to Fast and Pray: because there will be nothing else that they can Do about it, since they are not Prepared for any Great Famine. However, as a "Last Minute Emergency," they could Join the Church of Jesus Christ of Latter-day Saints, who Supposedly have a 7-Year Supply of Foods Stored Up for their own People.

18-04 [_] Nevertheless, you cannot Count on it: because Mormons have been known to LIE; but, for Sure, the Mormons do not have a 7-Year Supply of WATER for each of their Members: because that would be more Water than is presently contained in all American Reservoirs, combined! That is, if they just continued to use Water like they are now using it, which is an Average of 120 Gallons per Day, per Person, which is about 919,800,000,000 Gallons of Water for 3 million People for 7 Years, or about one-hundredth enough Water for Americans, without using Water for Irrigating the Great Plains and the whole Eastern United States, which Relies on Rainwater. In other words, we Americans would have to Drastically Revise our Lifestyles, and even SHUT OFF our Toilets, Lawn Sprinklers, Car Washes, Laundromats, and Daily Showers, in Order to Survive such a Great Drought, if it did not Rain for 3.5 Years, as it is Prophesied in *Revelation 11,* which stands a Good Chance of being True.

— Chapter 19 —

Supplemental Thoughts

19-01 [_] From Time to Time someone may Add Supplemental Thoughts to this Book, if they are Required. In the Meantime, TRY your Best to Follow the Proper RULES for FASTING: so that your Mind is somewhat Enlightened by what you Experience, and Remember that it has been many Years since I had to Administer an Enema to myself: beCause I have Access to Fresh Immature Coconut Water, which Flushes Out the Bowels from the Top Down, and without any Gases, Bloating, nor even an Uncomfortable Feeling: beCause it is the Perfect Flush, and especially for Old People. However, to be more Aggressive about Removing the Sticky Filth within a Person, such Immature Coconut Water needs some Lime Juice in it, which may Cause a little Bloating. Just be Sure to Drink Enough to get a Good Reaction from it — such as a Half Gallon or more of Immature Coconut Water, depending on how Long it has been since you Flushed Out your Bowels. And yes, it is Expensive; but, so are the Services of Medical Doctors by a hundred to a thousand Times!

19-02 [_] If you are Desperate for a Good Quiet Place to do your Fasting, you might try Contacting **The Worldwide People's Revolution!®**

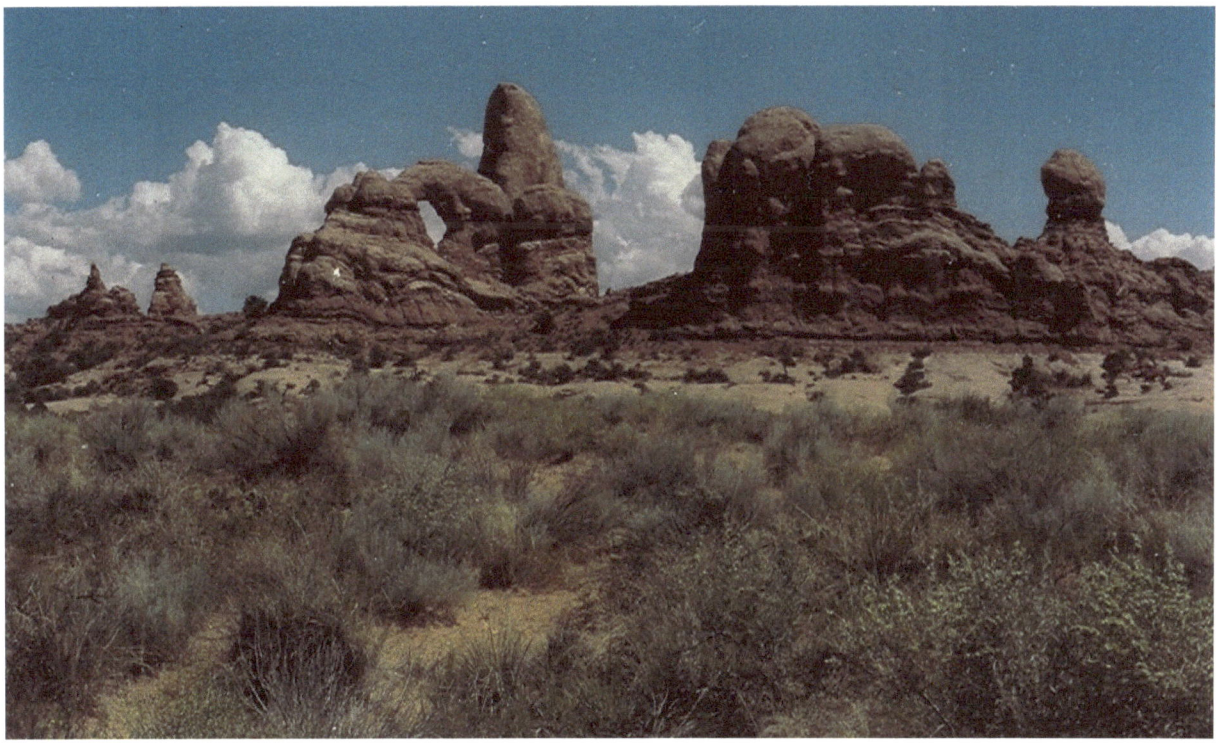

{FOOTNOTE: You might Think that this would be an Ideal Place to Fast and Pray, in Arches National Park, in Utah; but, rest assured, you would soon be Discovered and Cast Out within a couple Weeks without Special Permission. Moreover, if you told them about Fasting, you can be

Sure that you would be Cast Out sooner than that, if you were not Locked up in some Insane Asylum! Therefore, be Extra Careful when Dealing with the Devil.}

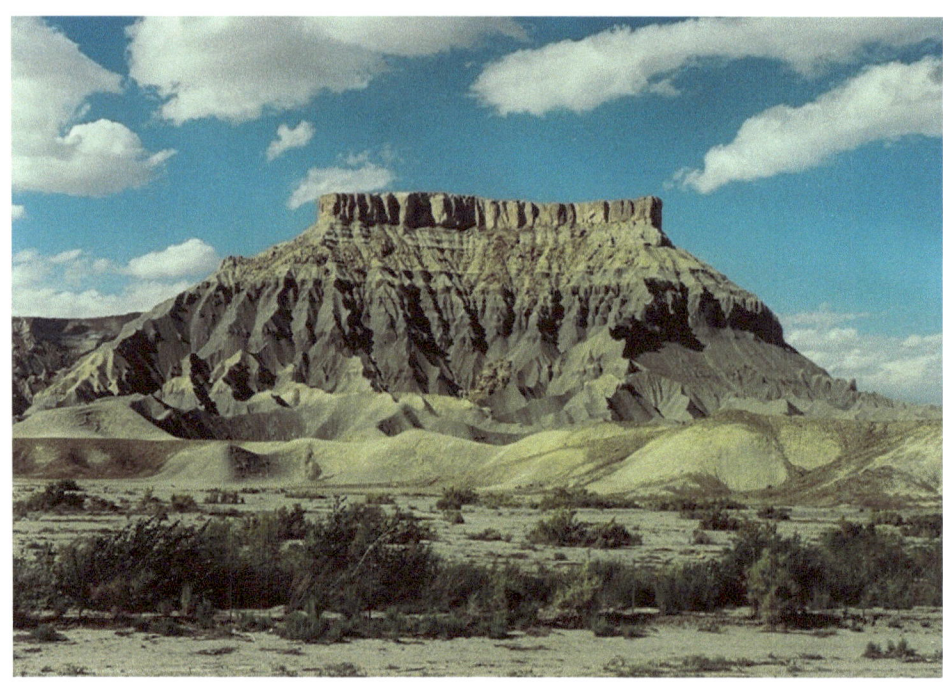

{FOOTNOTE: Now, you might Imagine that this would be an Ideal Place to Fast and Pray with Moses, Elijah, Alma, or Abinadi; but, behold, it gets very Cold at Night, which can make it very Uncomfortable, if not Deadly. Moreover, getting yourself Up on Top of that Butte with a couple Jugs of Spring Water, Prune Juice, Fresh Orange Juice, Coconut Water, Tent, Backpack with Tools, and everything you Need for Success, could prove to be almost Impossible, even with the Help of Joshua, Elisha, or some other Humble and Obedient Servant. Nevertheless, if I were the Elected King, we could Build a Proper Swanky Fasting Sanitarium not far from where I took the Photograph, and that would make it Practical for Fasting.}

— Chapter 20 —

A List of other Fascinating Literature by the same Inspired Author

20-001 [_]"LIGHTNING Versus the Lightning Bug!" (HOW almost Everyone can become Moderately RICH, without Telling Any Lies nor Selling Any Trash!) By The Worldwide People's Revolution!® Book 001. The Cover Photo shows a Beautiful Sunrise in the Blest Land of Eternal Springtime, where the little Birds of Cheerfulness are Singing, and the Fragrant Flowers are Blooming on the Trees of Life!

20-002 [_] "What is WRong with those Professing Christians?" (A Self-Examination of the Heart of the Body of Good Government!) By The Worldwide People's Revolution!® The Cover Photo shows a Small Portion of our Retirement Home. Many Photos with Explanations can be found Inside of the Books, just as soon as I can get them Updated. Please be Patient. Meanwhile, be Wise, and get yourself some Collector's Items: beCause these are very HOT Books, which you can Discover by Reading: **"The IDEAL Place to Live!"** Book 069.

20-003 [_] "For the Love of Money!" (The Strange Things that People Say and Do to Get more Money!) The Cover Photo shows a Jewish Boy Studying the *Scriptures.* Wise People do it all of the Time; but, some go Crazy for the Love of Money!

20-004 [_] "HOW to Prepare for CLIMATE CHANGES!" (The Wisest Plan for Mankind to Follow!) The Cover Photo shows Dark Awesome Clouds.

20-005 [_] "WHY do I have to be Surrounded by CRAZY PEOPLE?" (Do almost all People Feel like they are Surrounded by CRAZY PEOPLE??) The Cover Photo shows Delicious Sweet Fragrant Ripe Mangos, which were Grown by: **"The LUSCIOUS All-Mineral Organic Method of Gardening!" (HOW to Grow DELICIOUS Satisfying Foods for Potential Kingz and Kweenz in Swanky PALACES!)** Book 021. †

20-006 [_] "The Washington Journal is a FARCE!" (C-SPAN Managers are not very WISE!) The Cover Photo shows a small Portion of Mars, up Close. This Book tells about Proper Courting, and a Chain of Command System, which also has lots of Humor for Entertainment. †

20-007 [_] "The PRAYERS of PUMPKINHEADS!" (Even God Needs a Little Humor to Cheer himself Up!) The Cover Photo shows the Author's Brother measuring a Tree.

20-008 [_] "A Sound Argument for Masters and Servants!" (WHY Everyone Needs a Good Master, and every Master Needs Good Obedient Servants!) The Cover Photo shows a Pleasant Manmade Waterfalls.

20-009 [_] "WHY are some Preachers so POOR?" (HOW almost all Preachers could Get Moderately RICH, without Preaching any Outlandish LIES!) The Cover Photo shows the Inside of a Gold-laden Church in the Blest Land of Eternal Springtime.

20-010 [_] "GOOD NEWS for REBEL WOMEN!" (HOW almost all Wives can become Moderately RICH without Leaving their Homes! Guaranteed!) The Cover Photo shows Beautiful Ceramic Work in the Blest Land of Eternal Springtime. Chapter 04 is Extremely Good.

20-011 [_] "The Low Court of Supreme Injustices is Brought to Trial!" (Our Elected King Butts Heads with the United States Supreme Court, with or without their Black Robes of Hypocrisies and Lies!) By The Worldwide People's Revolution!® The Cover Photo shows the U.S. Supreme Court Building. This Special Book contains the Famous *Declaration of Interdependence,* and the Correct Wording for the Placard on the Statue of Liberty.

20-012 [_] "The Right Design for Living!" (A List of Great Advantages for Building Beautiful Planned City States!) The Cover Photo shows the Great Pyramid at Chichen Itza, in Mexico. There are also many Photos of Swanky Mulching Rocks and other Good Things.

20-013 [_] "The Gospel According to our Elected King!" (The Good News from the Most Modern Perspective!) The Cover Photo shows a very Dirty Drunkard lying by the Street. This Book contains the NMV of Jonah's Sermon, and the Story of the Prodigal Son.

20-014 [_] "Poverty Hunger Riots Strikes Brutalities Election Deceptions and Civil Wars!" (The High Price that we Earthlings have Paid for Leaving the Good Land!) The Cover Photo shows Tombs in a Cemetery. This Inspired Book deals with a Host of Important Subjects.

20-015 [_] "Seven Great Armies of Working Soldiers!" (HOW to Provide a Way for Everyone to WORK: so as to Eliminate Poverty, Crimes, Drug Abuses, Prisons and Unnecessary Taxes!) The Cover Photo shows a Truckload of Potential Working Soldiers. This Book tells about one of my True Life Stories when I was in the Army.

20-016 [_] "The CONSTITUTION for the New RIGHTEOUS One-World GovernMINT!" (HOW all Peoples can get True Justice, and Celebrate the Great Year of JUBILEE!) The Cover Photo shows a Gathering Thunderstorm. This Book presents the 9/11/2001 Case, Grades and Bonds.

20-017 [_] "The Great World TEMPLE of PEACE!" (The Glory of Jerusalem Arises Again!) By The Worldwide People's Revolution!® The Cover Photo shows Old Jerusalem.

20-018 [_] "The Swanky Associations of Working Soldiers!" (A Fascinating Collection of Various Kinds of Voluntary Working Soldiers!) The Cover Photo shows a Malachite Pyramid. This Book is for Adults, only.

20-019 [_] "GLORIOUS Swanky Hotels Castles and Fortresses!" (Beautiful Planned City States for WISE Intelligent Well-Educated People with Common Sense and Good

Understanding!) The Cover Photo shows a Beautiful "Million-dollar" Onyx Box. This Book tells about Abraham's Tomb and the Samson Story.

20-020 [_] **"Are you a Jobless Graduate of the SKQL uv FQLZ?" (HOW to Get a GOUD EJUKAASHUN without Robbing the Bank!)** The Cover Photo shows a small and Beautiful Onyx Vase. The Book contains the NMV of *First Corinthians 13,* and Describes Living Water.

20-021 [_] **"The LUSCIOUS All-Mineral Organic Method of Gardening!" (HOW to Grow DELICIOUS Satisfying Foods for Potential Kingz and Kweenz in Swanky PALACES!)** The Cover Photo shows Beautiful Green Terraces. The Book contains many Photos with Explanations for our 100,000-gallon Cistern for Water Storage, which took 7 Years to Build.

20-022 [_] **"Did God or Satan Ordain Medical Doctors??" (Ask Huck Finn and/or Nigger Jim: because neither Tom Sawyer nor Judge Thatcher would Know!)** The Cover Photo shows Pretty Flowers at a Tomb. This Book contains the New MAGNIFIED Version (NMV) of John 3, which is very Enlightening to the Mind of Greater Faith.

20-023 [_] **"The BIG White OUTHOUSE on the Not-so-Biblical Capitol DUNGHILL!" (The Chief Sins of the Divided States of United Lies!)** The Cover Photo shows the Capitol Building in the District of Corruption, in Washington.

20-024 [_] **"The Public School of IGNERUNT FQLZ!" (HOW we have been GRAATLEE DISEEVD!)** The Cover Photo shows a Disorganized Fruit Market in a City of Confusion.

20-025 [_] **"In thu Beeginingz uv Thingz!" (Thu Kreeaashun Stooree frum thu Beegining!)** The Cover Photo shows a Yellow / Golden Sapote, which not one Person in a Million in America has ever Tasted, in spite of being one of the most Pleasant Sweetest Fruits known to Mankind, which does not Ship Well, which must be Ripened on the Tree, to be Extremely GOOD! †

20-026 [_] **"God Speaks and the Whole World Listens!" (Fire on the Mountain from the Burning Bush by the Spirit of Truth!)** The Cover Photo shows the Sign or Flag for: **"The New RIGHTEOUS One-World Government!"** This Book contains the Best Noah Stories.

20-027 [_] **"Does a Good Soldier have to be a MURDERER?" (Seven Great Swanky Armies of Voluntary Working Soldiers!)** The Cover Photo shows Danny Boy.

20-028 [_] **"Thu Nq MAGNUFIID Verzhun uv Thu PROVERBZ uv KING SOLUMUN in Plaan Ingglish!" (The Understandable Version of the Famous Proverbs of King Solomon in Plain English!)** The Cover Photo shows my Gemstones in an Onyx Jewelry Box.

20-029 [_] **"UNLIMITED ENERJEE 99 Percent Pollutions Free!" (HOW to Obtain FREE ElecTrickery, Worldwide!)** The Cover Photo shows an Onyx Tray for a large Spoon.

20-030 [_] **"FREEDUM uv SPEECH!" (U Speshoul Maguzeen uv Onist Upinyunz!)** The Cover Photo shows a Portion of one of the Author's Marble Countertops, worth 100$ per square foot, for an Example of what you could also have, if you Exercised your Faith, Hope, Trust,

Love, Patience, Persistence, and OBEDIENCE! This Book Lists the Advantages for using Swanky Mulching Rocks, and Explains Baptism by Fire and Speaking in Tongues.

20-031 [_] "A Sure Cure for GUN VIOLENCE!" (HOW TO STOP GANG WARS and CRIMINAL SHOOTINGS!) The Cover Photo shows a Short Shotgun.

20-032 [_] "AIIRMWVC and Reasonable Solutions!" (Aliens, Illegal Immigrants, Refugees, Migrant Workers and other Victims of Capitalism!) The Cover Photo shows a "Sea of People." This Book contains the NMV of Jobe 33.

20-033 [_] "Mark Twain Races for the PRESIDENCY!" (The 2020 Presidential Candidates Desperately Need Some STRONG Undefeatable COMPETITION!) The Cover Photo shows a Mountain Goat and a Silver Dollar. This Book contains my Surveys of Values, plus several Photos of Union Station and Monuments in Washington, D.C.

20-034 [_] "ECCLESIASTES UNCOVERED!" (The New MAGNIFIED Version of Ecclesiastes and the Song of Solomon in Plain English!) The Cover Photo shows a Peacock.

20-035 [_] "The Environmentalists' Paradise!" (HOW almost Everyone could be Living in a Beautiful Manmade Paradise!) The Cover Photo shows an Artist's Conception of Paradise for a single Family in the Blest Land of Perfect Oneness. The Book contains the NMV of Psalm 48 in Plain English.

20-036 [_] "The Seven Basic Spiritual Building Blocks of LIFE!" (Faith Hope Trust Love Patience Persistence and Obedience!) The Cover Photo shows Onion Domes trimmed with Gold. This Book contains the Mockingbird's Version of Hebrews 11, plus 1st Corinthians 13.

20-037 [_] "DIETS!" (A Reasonable Solution for the "Eternal Controversy"!) The Cover Photo shows some Colorful Fruits.

20-038 [_] "The Nature of CAPITALISM!" (A List of the EVILS of CAPITALISM!) This Book will contain many Photos with Explanations when it gets Updated. The Cover Photo shows a pretty Red Car. If you discover other Photos in the Book, it means that it has been Updated.

20-039 [_] "SWANGKEENOMIKS Rules the Roost!" (HOW all People can Prosper in a RIIT WAA, and STOP Polluting the Earth with Capitalist TRASH!) The Cover Photo shows a small Portion of our Retirement Home, before the 5,000+ sq. ft. Roof was Installed.

20-040 [_] "The New MAGNIFIED Version of The Book of MOORMUN!" (The Story of the White and Dark Indians in the Americas!) The Cover Photos for Volumes 1 & 2 show the Queen of England's Golden Coach, and one of our Marbleous Spanish Walls, which is Worth a thousand dollars per square yard, which is installed on 7 Walls.

20-041 [_] "The Great Worldwide TELEVISED Court HEARING!" (That Great Meeting of the Most Intelligent Minds!) The Cover Photo shows Mount Popotits covered with Snow.

20-042 [_] "The Secret City of the Great King!" (HOW the True Church will Escape from the Great Tribulation!) The Cover Photo shows a Colorful Ferris Wheel. P-5877. You can expect many Photos to be Inside of the Book during the Future.

20-043 [_] "Terrorists Beware that your Days are Numbered!" (HOW to Bring those Terrorist Attacks to a Screeching HALT!) The Cover Photo shows a Picture of George Warmonger Bush. This Book also contains the Fascinating Book of LEHI, which was Lost since the 1830's! †

20-044 [_] "The New MAGNIFIED Version of ISAIAH in Plain English!" (The Understandable Version of the Book of Isaiah!) The Cover Photo shows a Swanky Potato / Avocado Salad with Sweet Peas, Corn, Shredded Carrots, Celery and Black Olives. This Book will soon contain many Photos of Agate Windows.

20-045 [_] "HOW to Become a HOLY Man!" (40 Good Reasons WHY People Should FAST and PRAY!) The Cover Photo will show the Face of a Holy Man, just as soon as one Presents himself for the Photograph.

20-046 [_] "The Proper RULES for FASTING!" (The Complete Instruction Manual for True Repentance!) The Cover Photo shows an Unclean Man. There are many Photos within this Book, already, including one of me with nothing but a Fig Leaf on for Clothing.

20-047 [_] "Are Americans the Most STUPID People who ever Lived?" (HOW Working People can PROSPER and Live in PEACE Under the Rulership of a RIGHTEOUS KING!) The Cover Photo shows a large Portion of the Author's Marbleous Living Room Floor.

20-048 [_] "An Amazing Collection of Wit and Wisdom!" (The Marvelous Tale of the Colorful Peacock from Angel Ridge, and the Strong Rope of Hope!) The Cover Photo shows a Book Display.

20-049 [_] "Justifications for Capitalizations!" (WHY our Elected King Defies the School of Fools by Capitalizing LOVE and HATE!) The Cover Photo shows a Water Tower.

20-050 [_] "The END of CONFUSION!" (The Great CELEBRATION of the Magnificent Wedding of the Humble Honest Nations, and the Grand Year of JUBILEE!) The Cover Photo shows a Portion of a Colorful Parade from an Eagle's Point of View.

20-051 [_] "The Loathsome Burdens of the Independent Jackasses!" (A New Approach for Solving our Massive Problems!) The Cover Photo shows a Spanish Military Barracks.

20-052 [_] "Are we Tax Slaves of a Lower Order than Lying Red JEWS?" (HOW to be Liberated from all Slavery, Worldwide!) The Cover Photo shows a few Tax Slaves.

20-053 [_] "The Great False Economy is now DEBUNKED!" (Adolf Hitler had a much Better Economic System!) The Cover Photo shows a Capitalist Toilet Brush.

20-054 [_] **"The UGLY Scarred Dishonest Face of Poor Old Miserable UNCLE SAM!" (A Memorial Day Legacy!)** The Cover Photo shows a Poster of "Uncle Sam," who Symbolizes the Federal Government of **"The Divided States of United Lies!" (The so-called "United States of North America" in Disguise!)**

20-055 [_] **"The United States of the Whole World!" (A True Global Economy for the Masses of Working People!)** The Cover Photo shows a 110-year-old Well-made Mexican Rocking Chair with a Cowhide Seat — that is, IF I can get my Computer to Working again.

20-056 [_] **"The New RIGHTEOUS One-World Government!" (HOW to Establish a Righteous One-World Government without Going to WAR!)** The Cover Photo shows the Flag or Sign for that Good Government.

20-057 [_] **"Those Ridiculous Contradictions within the Holy Bible!" (HOW to Read the Bible with an Open Mind!)** The Cover Photo shows a Thorny Rose Bush.

20-058 [_] **"The Divided States of United Lies!" (The so-called "United States of North America" in Disguise!)** The Cover Photo shows a Map of the United States.

20-059 [_] **"The Complete SURVEYS of our VALUES!" (SURVEYS of Religious Spiritual Political Governmental Sexual Social Moral Economic Business Labor Habitual and Miscellaneous VALUES!)** The Cover Photo shows a large Onyx Vase in the Author's Palace.

20-060 [_] **"HOW to Get our PRIORITIES in ORDER!" (The Glories of Democracy; and, Does DEMON-ocracy have its Priorities in Order?)** The Cover Photo shows a Different View of that Onyx Vase.

20-061 [_] **"The New MAGNIFIED Version of the GOOD NEWS According to Saint LUKE!" (The Magnified Gospel of Luke in Plain English!)** The Cover Photo shows some Agate Windows. Many more Beautiful Photos can be seen within that Exceptionally Good Book.

20-062 [_] **"The New MAGNIFIED Version of the GOOD NEWS According to Saint JOHN!" (The Gospel According to Saint John Zebedee Boanerges in Plain English!)** The Cover Photo shows the Parthenon.

20-063 [_] **"The New MAGNIFIED Version of the Book of ACTS!" (The Understandable Version of the ACTS of the Apostles in Plain English!)** The Cover Photo shows a Small Portion of Arches National Park, in Utah, the Headquarters of the Latter-day Sinners!

20-064 [_] **"The New MAGNIFIED Version of the PSALMS of King David!" (The Understandable Version of the Famous Psalms in Plain English!)** The Cover Photo shows some of the Grand Canyon.

20-065 [_] **"A List of FAIR Swanky Wages!" (The Equitable Wage System!)** The Cover Photo shows a Pile of Money. This Book contains the Famous Poem, called: "HOW could we Afford it?" You will no doubt Love it.

20-066 [_] **"Beautiful Swanky PALACES!" (A New Concept in Living Habits — Swanky Palaces for Poor People!)** The Cover Photo shows a Bouquet of Pretty Flowers in my Kitchen.

20-067 [_] **"The Swanky Sword of Divine Truths!" (The Most Powerful Weapon in the Whole Universe!)** The Cover Photo shows a Lazy Robe with a Split Sword.

20-068 [_] **"Has your Life become Extremely Complicated?" (HOW to Live a SIMPLE Life!)** The Cover Photo shows a Retired Race Horse.

20-069 [_] **"The IDEAL Place to Live!" (HOW to Discover an Ideal Place to Live!)** The Cover Photo shows an Ideal Place to Live. This Book contains at least 66 Photographs with Explanations for your Enlightenment.

20-070 [_] **"Our Elected King Who Speaks Out!" (It is High Time for some Sane Person to Get Control of this Insane World!)** The Cover Photo shows a Part of New York City from the Top of the Empire State Building.

20-071 [_] **"How GAY is GOD?" (Oh the Wonders of it all when it ALL Hangs Out!)** The Cover Photo shows some Unbelievable Private Parts!

The Enticement,

Our Elected King, has undertaken many hundreds of Fasts during his Lifetime — the Longest being 314 Days during 14 Months, after which he was as Strong as Samson, you might say. The Great Shame of it all was the Fact that he was too Poor at the Time to Afford to Eat Good Healthy Foods, whereby he might have Maintained such a Wonderful State of Good Health. Indeed, his Naaberz only Envied him for it, and Refused to Assist him in any Way, which is likely what you will also Discover, if you do a LOT of Fasting and Praying: beCause Satan, himself, will be Against you, which Means that all False Churches will also be Against you! Nevertheless, **The Worldwide People's Revolution!®** Hopes to Change all of that.